# Dragon
Within the Gates

# Dragon
## Within the Gates

*The Once and Future AIDS Epidemic*

Stephen C. Joseph, M.D.

Carroll & Graf Publishers, Inc.
New York

Copyright © 1992 by Stephen C. Joseph, M.D.

First Carroll & Graf edition 1992

Carroll & Graf Publishers, Inc.
260 Fifth Avenue
New York, NY 10001

Library of Congress Cataloging-in-Publication Data is available.

ISBN: 0-88184-905-7

Manufactured in the United States of America

FOR E.A.P.

# Acknowledgments

A number of organizations and individuals contributed in diverse ways to the writing of this book.

The following foundations provided generous support which enabled the author to undertake the work: The Commonwealth Fund, The Robert Wood Johnson Foundation, The Henry J. Kaiser Family Foundation, The Josiah Macy, Jr., Foundation, and The New York Community Trust.

The assistance of the United Hospital Fund and its President, Bruce Vladeck, is also gratefully acknowledged.

My patient agent, Theron Raines, and Julia Vitullo-Martin, who edited an early draft of the manuscript, were valued guides.

I am indebted to former colleagues at the New York City Department of Health, whose professionalism is too seldom recognized by the public they serve.

All opinions, and any errors of fact or omission, are, of course, completely the author's responsibility.

Because my intent is to make this book widely accessible to the general public, scientific terminology and complexity have been simplified, in some instances, for purposes of greater clarity.

# Contents

# Introduction: African Genesis

Epidemic: a disease prevalent among a people or a community at a special time, and produced by some special causes not generally present in the affected society

*Oxford English Dictionary*
*From the Greek roots epi* (upon or among) and *demos* (the people); literally *upon the people*

Some years into the future, we will come to realize that despite the devastating effects of AIDS as one of the twentieth century's major epidemics, we were more fortunate than we might have been; it could well have been worse.

It is difficult for us to comprehend this now, in the midst of the epidemic's first explosive phase. It will be easier to understand later, when the fires burn lower. By the adult years of our grandchildren, when the virus reaches its long accommodation with society, we will see clearly that despite the enormous toll in death and disability, the epidemic might indeed have hit harder.

AIDS might have been caused by a virus much more easily transmissible among people, and less selective in its modes of spread. It might have had an even longer silent period of latency between infection and disease, thus making more difficult our understanding of cause and effect. And, had the epidemic appeared even twenty years earlier, we would not have had the tools of basic science with which so rapidly to identify, characterize, and begin to combat the infectious agent. Thus, AIDS might have spread more rapidly and generally, remained more inscrutable, and been even less subject to our prevention and treatment efforts than it has.

AIDS will not account for anything near the short-term intensity of illness and death of this century's other major worldwide epidemics. The 1918 influenza epidemic alone killed more than ten million people in four years. Neither will AIDS have the sustained high toll garnered by the twentieth century's major epidemics of behavior: coronary artery disease, lung cancer, and motor vehicle accidents.

Will AIDS, when viewed from a future retrospective, match the societal devastation of the great plagues of ancient and medieval times? It is highly unlikely that this will be so for the United States and other affluent countries, but the true scale of the tragedy now developing in Africa and elsewhere in the Third World is not yet accurately predictable. We tend to forget that the great plagues of former times were not so much "events" as processes, often stretching over decades in waves of infection. Viewed from that perspective, AIDS may indeed take greater prominence.

Yet AIDS has a special importance and intensity. It is a characteristically twentieth-century epidemic: it is both a pandemic (worldwide epidemic) infection attacking societies that had just begun to believe themselves invulnerable to mass infectious disease, and it is an epidemic closely related to current behavior. Despite this very contemporary character, the virus's sexual and drug connections call forth the deepest psychic responses much as the great medieval plagues did.

In one sense, the first years of the AIDS epidemic were reminiscent of the conceptions of epidemics portrayed in Greek tragedies: a mysterious agent sweeps through groups of "outsiders"; it is associated with taboo behaviors; it gives no sign of its presence until the person afflicted becomes ill with an ultimately fatal wasting disease; there is no clear explanation of this previously unknown phenomenon; there is no recovery, no treatment, and no cure.

But from another perspective, AIDS is the first truly modern epidemic, and presages important trends for future epidemics and other major health issues. Its definition in political and social terms, the astonishing speed with which basic science and applied medicine and public health began to solve its riddles, the powerful distrust of government and health institutions on the part of those most affected by the epidemic, and the power of its victims in shaping the entire social response: these are quite new and contemporary phenomena.

Also emblematic of its modernity is the fact that the major modes of spread involve voluntary and conscious behaviors (principally sexual and drug-using behaviors), and that the initial approaches to prevention of further spread involved attempts to persuade people to modify that voluntary behavior.

Because AIDS is so closely related to behavior, because it is a worldwide pandemic of infection coming at a time when we had begun to believe that we were no longer vulnerable to mass infectious disease, and because the sexual and drug connections of the human immunodeficiency virus call forth our deepest psychic responses in the way the great plagues of antiquity and the Middle Ages must have done in their own time: for all these reasons, AIDS has taken a special importance and a special intensity of meaning.

There is a balance here between the pain, loss, rage, frustration, and costs on one end of the scale, and the lessons to be learned, the applicable knowledge to be gained, and the realization that it might have been much worse on the other end of the scale. That balance, so heavily weighted against us, is cold comfort now. But our great-great-grandchildren, who will not truly feel our pain or sense of loss, will look with more objectivity at both ends of the scale.

This book gives a perspective on the first decade of AIDS, and then projects into the decade to come. It emphasizes in detail the public health and public policy issues in New York City, at the epicenter of the first decade of the North American AIDS epidemic. It speaks of the major opportunities, repeatedly missed, to take strong public health stands to protect against further spread of the virus, to prevent (or at least to ameliorate) a second wave of infection among minority women and children. The book warns that the sharp impact of death and disease from this virus is still ahead, and that there is greater urgency than ever to take the preventive actions that can protect the uninfected. The human immunodeficiency virus must be seen as a living organism with any species' innate drive for survival and increase: it cannot be combated with hope and rhetoric, but only by building obstacles to its transmission and survival.

Those necessary obstacles involve both the alteration of individual behavior, and the public health protection of communities.

New York City was, and is, the site that exemplified the power of the epidemic: its relentless rise to over 40,000 cases and over 25,000 deaths in the city within the space of a decade; its corrosive impact on already hard-pressed medical and social services; its increasing focus (as with most epidemics) on poor and minority populations; and above all its ability to ignite bitter social conflict. In these respects, AIDS further recalls the great plagues of classical and medieval times, and the City of New York was where this drama was most sharply silhouetted.

With the virus already very widely seeded within high-risk groups (homosexual and bisexual men, and intravenous drug users), my years of direct involvement as New York City's Commissioner of Health (1986–1990) saw the explosion of clinical illness and deaths, the broader emergence of heterosexual transmission and its effects on black and Hispanic women and children, the new linkage of AIDS with the crack/cocaine epidemic, and the accompanying wide-ranging political and ethical controversies. These years also crystallized the search for appropriate public health responses to and containment of the epidemic. This early response was shaped by strongly held and strongly conflicting attitudes, both public and professional.

To understand where we are in this epidemic and where we should go, we need to begin at the beginning. As with the emergence of the human species, and as with many, perhaps most, of the illnesses that have accompanied the human journey, so it was with the origin of AIDS: in Africa.

The virus that causes AIDS, the human immunodeficiency virus or HIV 1, first gained a foothold in humans some fifty or more years ago in Africa. Transmuted from a simian virus, it leaped to humans, most probably to hunters and their families who killed, gutted, and ate the monkeys countless times and in countless places in East and Central Africa. For most of that half-century, the virus was unrecognized and quiescent, perhaps a low-virulence progenitor to the current strain, more probably seeping slowly through rural Africa, with the illness undiagnosed and unnamed.

I remember a number of patients, adults and children, during the early 1970s when I practiced medicine in Central Africa, patients with wasting syndromes, atypical progressive infections, bizarre malignancies—all undiagnosed due to lack of laboratory facilities or lack of specific knowledge.

I had gone to work for the A.I.D. (Agency for International Development) in Cameroon, where an international consortium was developing a new medical school based on community medicine principles. As part of my work with the medical school, I ran the young children's ward at the local capital city hospital. I supervised a ward of fifty to sixty children under five years of age, all of whom were desperately ill. There were children dying of malaria, measles, meningitis, polio, pneumonia, diarrhea, and dehydration. Beneath these illnesses, the children almost invariably suffered from severe malnutrition. The death rate was consistently high—15 percent of all the children on my ward died.

Most of the mortally ill children I was caring for had a combination of severe malnutrition and one or more infectious diseases. These children were in a way the analog to today's people with AIDS—they suffered malnutrition to such an extreme that their immune systems collapsed. Were some of these patients actually unrecognized cases of the wasting syndrome caused by infection with the human immunodeficiency virus, of the syndrome we would today call AIDS? We do know that some human blood samples drawn in East and West Africa in the 1960s and 1970s apparently contained antibodies to the human immunodeficiency virus, though the specificity of this has been challenged.

It is likely that, across the broad central belt of Africa, hundreds, perhaps thousands, of adults and children died of HIV infection prior to the 1970s, unattended by modern medicine, or undiagnosed as anything other than the common pattern of Third World overwhelming infection and malnutrition.

The virus lingered, waiting for its moment, and then exploded in the 1970s, with a rapid outflow of infection through Africa, in the Caribbean, in North America, and in Europe. Because it usually takes at least three to five years after infection with the virus to develop full-blown AIDS, and because the first clinical cases were recognized in the United States (in Los Angeles and New York) in 1981, followed by rapid recognition of increasingly large numbers of AIDS cases in many other countries over the next year or two, we also know that the first period of rapid spread had to be in the late 1970s—not earlier and not later. Why this breakout fifty years or more after the virus first gained a foothold in humans? Why then, and not before?

History demonstrates that an epidemic's creation requires not only the microbe but also the appropriate social context. War, major population movements, natural disasters and climatic or environmental changes, marked shifts in cultural patterns—all have been traditional factors in creating and sustaining epidemics. The larger environment, its social patterns especially, is an indispensable ingredient in the where and when of epidemics.

As in the ancient image of the horsemen of the Apocalypse—War, Famine, Pestilence, and the Pale Rider, Death—the interactions of rapid social disorganization are the chief breeding grounds of epidemics. But any rapid or wholesale social change can alter the balance that keeps an infectious organism in check, or that provides a new setting which allows the emergence of a previously unknown threat.

Populations with no prior experience of a given infecting organism, with no prior history of individual immunity gained through proximity, are most vulnerable to an explosive and highly fatal epidemic when a new invader appears, especially if the social environment is simultaneously destabilized.

The microbe does not act alone.

Two especially instructive African examples are the sleeping sickness epidemics of the nineteenth century and the cholera epidemic of the 1970s. African sleeping sickness, a progressive, fatal disease in humans caused by a protozoan, with wild hoofed-mammals as hosts and the tsetse fly as a carrier, had existed in endemic form in Africa for centuries. But in the nineteenth century, horrific epidemics of sleeping sickness cut swathes through East and Central Africa (in many of the very same geographic areas where AIDS is now most prevalent), with thousands of cases and the virtual depopulation of whole villages and regions as people died or fled. These disease

outbreaks were themselves the outcomes of major social and geographic dislocations resulting from the slaving wars of the preceding
hundred years. One has only to read the journals of the colonial
military physicians to get a sense of the havoc and terror that the
sleeping sickness epidemics caused. These epidemics were themselves both the cause and the result of massive social destabilization:
the fearsome epidemics tore the normal fabric of village life apart;
the epidemics were the product of war's destruction of that fabric.

Asiatic cholera has its ancestral home in the riverine estuaries of
East Bengal. Though it has broken out many times in history and
spread widely around the world, it had never been reported from
the west coast of Africa. However, in the late 1960s and early 1970s,
a strain of cholera named El Tor broke out of Bangladesh, spread
across the Indian Ocean, Iran, the Middle East, across the Mediter-
ranean and North Africa and, for the first time, around the western
bulge of Africa, along the coast and into the interior.

I was living and working in Africa at the time. The speed with
which the disease progressed was impressive. On an almost daily
basis, we could follow the course of new appearances in port cities
and country after country by reading the *International Herald Trib-
une*. Within weeks of the cholera's first appearance in Nigerian
ports, we were grappling with widespread outbreaks in the villages
of the Chadian Sahel, a thousand miles inland.

As with the sleeping sickness epidemics of the century before,
and as with the medieval plagues in Europe, entire villages were
burned and abandoned by their terrified inhabitants, who fled, taking the infection with them to surrounding districts. As Chadian and
French military units attempted to construct a "cordon sanitaire"
with (largely ineffective) vaccine, they were hard pressed to stay
ahead of the depopulated areas. In an impromptu field hospital,
constructed of thatched mats with patients laid in the sand, in the
first two weeks we treated adults critically ill with cholera. By the
third week, we were seeing increasing numbers of dehydrated and
malnourished infants, whose mothers had died of cholera in the first
two weeks.

Why cholera in West Africa in 1970 and never before? The answer lies less in the variety of the microbe than in the impact of

modern transportation patterns: by air, across sea lanes, and by new road and truck travel to the interior; and in the rapid urbanization of newly independent African states, with urban coastal crowding, mass poverty, unsafe water supplies, and inadequate waste disposal systems.

The spread of cholera to West Africa in the 1970s was, in part, an epidemic caused by what we could term "progress"—the globalization of rapid transportation and trade—and in part an epidemic based on the traditional factors of poverty and lack of sanitation.

Lest anyone think that this cholera example is a chapter of the past, there is a similar cholera epidemic spreading northward and eastward from recent outbreaks in the South American Andes. In early 1992, five passengers on a 330-person jet arriving in Los Angeles were stricken with cholera, and at least twenty-five more were found to be infected. The infection was subsequently traced to contaminated food boarded onto the plane either in Buenos Aires or Lima.

The 1970s African cholera story has a coda, one that along with the importance of rapid modern transport and urban agglomeration has a powerful message for the future of AIDS. Once the cholera bacterium reached the coastal rivers of West Africa, where it had never been before, it found an ecologic welcome. It settled in and persists today in estuaries all along the West African coast. Since that initial epidemic of the early 1970s, it surges inland again from time to time, in response to who knows what combination of human and environmental circumstances, creating recurrent local epidemics. These localized outbreaks do not have the virulence or the mass mortality of the initial assault upon a previously unacquainted population, but cholera is installed in West Africa, for the long haul.

Why do the successive waves of an epidemic, particularly when a given disease is new to a population, generally exhibit less dramatic effect over time? Two reasons provide at least partial explanation. First, as with any predator/prey relationship, a new disease-causing agent first selects the most vulnerable subjects, the ones most likely to be attacked, and the ones least able to resist. Second, with a new disease, the most extreme and dramatic forms are recognized initially; as time goes on, less florid, less lethal, less typical examples become part of the diagnostic pattern.

Both these factors have important implications for the AIDS epidemic, and would lead us to predict a long persistence of new infections, a gradual broadening of the population groups affected, and a widening range of symptoms and degrees of illness recognized as being caused by the HIVirus.

At the beginning of our recognition of AIDS, in 1981, our horizon was limited to only five gay men in Los Angeles who were found to have a puzzling combination of (then) very rare symptoms that later came to be labeled "full-blown AIDS." Rapidly, clinicians and public health workers discovered larger and larger numbers of "people with AIDS," all of whom were dreadfully ill, all of whom were soon to die of their illness. The next stage of our awareness was that this illness which we called AIDS was really the end stage of a years' long process of infection with a human immunodeficiency virus, an infection that began silently years before the patient had any recognizable symptoms or indeed any knowledge that he had been infected.

Eventually, we came to recognize that infection with the human immunodeficiency virus (HIV) led progressively to an entire spectrum of illness, ranging from "mere" laboratory test abnormalities in an otherwise well-appearing person, to a wide range of minor and major symptoms of ill health, to a diverse array of infections that attacked the immunocompromised host (the so-called opportunistic infections) and that were the clinical bellwethers of underlying infection with HIV, to a series of cancers also associated with HIV infection, and to, probably eventually in all HIV-infected individuals, the clinical pattern we initially had recognized as "AIDS."

Before too much longer, scientists will probably not use the term "AIDS" to describe this spectrum and this process. Rather, they will talk of "HIV Disease" and label its various stages by the degrees of failure of the immune system and the association of types of infection and cancer. We will see HIV infection for what it really is: a continuum, and one that runs a long drawn-out course of ten years or more between infection and death.

As with cholera and sleeping sickness, the human immunodeficiency virus found the appropriate human and natural circumstances for rapid spread and breakout in Africa in the 1970s. In the preceding two decades, the regions where the AIDS virus was seeded had undergone localized bursts of urbanization, and more generalized rapid population growth, social disorganization, famines, wars and civil conflicts (such as the successive wars in the then-Congo and in Uganda, two of the areas of the highest prevalence of AIDS early in the epidemic). This period also saw the development of modern road transport penetrating deep into rural interiors (in the Ugandan/Tanzanian AIDS epidemic, long distance truckers, soldiers, and roadside prostitutes who serviced both groups created the rural-to-urban passage of the virus).

In the new cities of Africa, social conditions were ripe for the spread of a sexually transmitted epidemic. Village and family structures had collapsed, poverty and prostitution were rampant, sanitation facilities largely nonexistent for the mass of the population, medical care inaccessible and inadequate, and effective public health education and control measures absent.

One of my colleagues, who ran the municipal sexually transmitted disease clinic in a Central African capital city, estimated in 1972 that at any one time 10 percent of the adult population of the city had gonorrhea.

Just as the virus found fertile ground in its passage from the African rural to urban areas, so the African urban settings provided a springboard to the rest of the world. The entry of Africa into global transportation and communications networks, the passages of European and Caribbean mercenary soldiers and military units, the emergence of large-scale tourism, the increased numbers of African students and business travelers in Europe and North America—all these were phenomena of the 1970s on a scale never before experienced by Africa. In addition, the growth of "sexual tourism" (homo-, hetero-, and bi-sexual) not only in Africa but also in Europe, North America, and the Caribbean basin, coincided with the availability of the virus for dissemination globally, and became a major feature of the earliest spread of the virus in and between the United States and Haiti.

Just how explosive the connection between prostitution and the

HIVirus can be—especially in settings where other sexually transmitted diseases are rampant and can make it easier for the HIVirus to gain entry to a new host through genital ulcers—was demonstrated during the first decade of the epidemic in East Africa by the rapid concentration of infection among urban prostitutes, and the subsequent dissemination of HIV infection through their male clients to their own wives in turn, so that by the decade's end the infection rate among women in several East African cities was shown to be in the range of 30 percent, an enormous figure in public health terms. In Africa, the rates of HIV infection are roughly equal between males and females, in keeping with the predominantly heterosexual nature of transmission, and in contrast to the much higher ratios of infected males to infected females in the United States in the first decade of the epidemic, reflecting homosexuality and intravenous drug injection as the predominant modes of spread.

Later, in 1991, in Thailand, the combination of sexual transmission and intravenous drug use among prostitutes, their pimps, and customers, led to the most explosive rate of HIV increase in prevalence yet recorded, going from virtually zero to the range of 50 percent infection rates among IV drug users and prostitutes within a two-year period. This example gives credence to the hypothesis that it had indeed been possible, in the years before the epidemic was recognized, for infection rates to climb from zero to 50 percent and 30 percent, respectively, among intravenous drug users and male homosexuals in New York City within a period of less than five years.

In Thailand, and in similar explosive rates of infection in the early stages of the epidemic now occurring in other developing countries in Asia and Latin America, we have had no greater success in applying those preventive measures that might have been adapted from the sad lessons of North America. For example, it might have been logical to view Thailand, with a large population of drug injectors, closely connected to a thriving sex industry that itself has pervasive international links, as inevitably ripe for an HIV explosion. What if clean needle availability and condom education (of both prostitutes and tourists) had been made major public health priorities in Thailand, along with a early-warning surveillance system for HIV infection in, say, 1988? Could the explosiveness of the epidemic have been muted? What about other countries in the world who "as yet have no AIDS problem" or, more accurately, have as yet failed to recognize that they have one, however incipient? Despite the expressions of public concern and the newspaper headlines, we seem to have failed as yet to grasp the major lesson of the epidemic: you are vulnerable before you realize you are vulnerable, and waiting until the dragon appears before taking every preventive action you can is to wait until too late.

We are so close to our own experience that it is difficult to get a good perspective on the mass movements, dislocations, and interconnections of the world's population in the twentieth century. Accelerating during and after the Second World War, these phenomena represent a major demographic event in world history, ranking with the Crusades, the European explorations and colonizations, and the earlier movements of Central Asian peoples into Europe. The current demographic super-event is distinguished both by very rapid population growth and by very large numbers of people on the move.

Every major historic demographic upheaval has had its accompanying plagues and epidemics, some remembered vividly, others lost in the mists. But the vivid, well-known examples—cholera, plague, and typhus brought to Europe during the Crusades; the sixteenth-century syphilis epidemic that swept Europe after importation from the New World; the virtual extermination of the peoples of North and South America and Oceania by common European diseases (such as measles) with which they had no prior experience—should leave us unsurprised that the twentieth century brings its own pattern of epidemics. The twentieth century is the century of global interconnection, and we should expect that major epidemics would be global—pandemics. And so they increasingly have been: typhus and influenza after the First World War, other global outbreaks (such as cholera) on a smaller scale, and now the first long-term, continuing, infectious disease pandemic: AIDS.

The AIDS virus broke out of Africa and, before we even knew of its existence, seeded heavily into other receptive environments:

New York and other American cities, Haiti, European capitals, and successively into other urban environments. With a perspective on the social and environmental context from which the epidemic arose, it seems it could not have been otherwise. It is when we come to discuss responding to the challenges that the epidemic continues to pose, that we will see how many might-have-beens there are.

As one realizes that this epidemic will burn its way across Africa for decades to come—even if effective treatment or a vaccine is found, unstoppable because of the poverty and fragile infrastructure of African nations and the inability and unwillingness of richer nations to come to their assistance—it is difficult to conceive of how the situation could be worse.

And yet, consider:

The Ebola virus was the cause of several epidemics of hemmorhagic fever in the southern Sudan and western Zaire in the 1970s, epidemics that caused thousands of deaths. A closely related virus (Marburg virus, which, like the specific Ebola strain, is not similar to any other known virus) caused a number of deaths in Europe in the late 1960s. Its entry was via infected African green monkeys which, imported into Europe, had infected laboratory workers handling blood and tissues. Other human contacts were then infected by transmission of human body fluids, including sexual transmission and aerosol spread (sneezing and coughing), and via contaminated needles and syringes. Mortality in the European cases was high, around 25 percent; mortality rates among the African cases are not known.

Another viral infection, Lassa fever, is widespread in Africa, and can cause a 15 percent or more mortality in hospitalized cases. It has been introduced into Europeans working as medical or research personnel in local African outbreaks, and is transmitted via direct contact with body fluids and secretions of a patient. Aerosol transmission is likely but unproven. Identification of a possible case in the United States calls forth emergency measures of isolation, disinfection of patient's excreta and articles with which the patient has been in contact, quarantine, and urgent tracing of contacts and possible sources of infection.

In the 1970s numerous localized outbreaks of infectious disease occurred in Africa, outbreaks that caused pockets of high death rates, but whose previously unknown viral agents were never able to ignite countrywide or worldwide self-sustaining epidemics.

Unlike the human immunodeficiency virus, the agents causing Ebola and Lassa fever disease, though they also cause very high mortality, are relatively easily transmitted from human to human, and result in illness within days or weeks.

Theoretically, a virus such as Lassa or Ebola should spread far more widely, and persist more easily than the human immunodeficiency virus, which is relatively inefficient in human-to-human transmission, has no other animal host, and cannot survive for any significant period outside the human body. Why AIDS and not a pandemic of Lassa fever, or of virus $x$? We will never know precisely, but the first lesson to be learned from the emergence of the AIDS pandemic is the lesson of human vulnerability.

With the sanitary revolution and the emergence of multiple vaccines and antimicrobial therapy, we came to believe in medicine's supposed conquest of mass infectious diseases. Infectious diseases in the privileged countries in the late twentieth century came to be thought of largely as issues fought out by doctors working with individual patients, mapped by sophisticated laboratory tests that probed even to subcellular levels. We began to delude ourselves that, at least in wealthy countries, plagues were things of the past.

AIDS has taught us that we are still vulnerable to the emergence of new or previously unrecognized agents capable of causing epidemic disease. In the globally interconnected context of our time and beyond, pandemics may actually become more likely. Next time, and there will surely be a next time, we may be less fortunate. The new agent might be capable of far more rapid spread, might be transmissible by a cough on the subway or the Concorde, might be capable of rapid mutation to stay ahead of whatever therapeutic miracles are next devised.

It is above all with a sense of human vulnerability and the frailty of human defenses that one recognizes some of the retrospective signposts of AIDS. One reads the account of the first physician presumed to have died after occupational exposure to the human immunodeficiency virus, a Danish surgeon exposed in Africa almost a decade before we recognized the first cases of AIDS in 1981; or of the Norwegian merchant seaman, his wife, and daughter, all of whom died of what clearly seems to have been AIDS in 1976, after illnesses that began in the late 1960s. What if this virus had been more readily communicable? What if there had been widespread and continuing infection with this fatal virus before we had developed the biologic sophistication adequate to clearly identify it?

When the world looks back on the biology of AIDS a hundred years hence, what will seem most remarkable will not be the way we stumbled in ignorance and confusion in the early years of the epidemic. Rather, the realization will be the precise opposite: how in five or ten very short years the knowledge base mushroomed— identification of the specific agent in less than three years, a reliable blood test for infection in four, detailed understanding of the biology of the virus and of its interaction with the human host cascading at an ever-increasing rhythm, the dawn of specific antiviral therapy within five years of identification of the virus, perhaps even a vaccine within fifteen or twenty years!

The AIDS epidemic links closely the two most important current frontiers of biomedicine: immunology and virology. The benefits that will flow—indeed are already flowing—from the new knowledge gained in attacking the AIDS puzzle will have stupendous and incalculable benefits in the research and application of tomorrow's biomedicine. For all the tragedy of AIDS, the potential gain of knowledge from the medical response to the epidemic also constitutes a moon-shot of enormous promise. The medical science of tomorrow will be able to treat infectious and chronic diseases that we are unable to treat today because of the greater understanding of how our immune systems react to stress and invasion. This knowledge will be applicable to the entire spectrum of illness; it will arise from what we learn from AIDS.

But what if the human immunodeficiency virus had arisen and broken out of Africa twenty or even fifteen years earlier? Medical knowledge of viruses, the immune system, molecular genetics, subcellular events, was relatively primitive just a short a time ago. We never could have recognized in biological detail, let alone been able to respond to, the AIDS challenge, had it burst upon us two decades earlier.

And so, out of Africa, the virus came to us. It was widely spread and entrenched in New York City and elsewhere well before we knew of its existence. The dragon was within the gates before we even knew it was coming, before the alarm could be sounded, let alone before preparations could be made for the city's defense. As Camus says in *The Plague:* "Wars and plagues are always with us, but equally they always take us by surprise."

# 1

## The Once and Future Epidemic

I WAS THE COMMISSIONER OF HEALTH OF NEW YORK CITY FROM 1986 to 1990, when New York became the epicenter of the AIDS epidemic in the United States. Those years saw both the full explosion of the epidemic and our gradual understanding of its nature. They were years of stridency and fear, sometimes of violence and terror, as the epidemic moved from its initial concentration among gay men to minority drug users of both sexes. Clashes of policy and politics about disease reporting and contact tracing, antibody testing, education of the public, distribution of needles and syringes to drug addicts, and the estimates of the extent of the epidemic itself became daily and troubling arguments.

In some ways this is a story of our society's failure—the failure to meet the challenges of the epidemic despite scientific accomplishments far beyond what might have been expected. Failures occurred in part because of the nature of the disease and in part because of social stigmas concerning the people initially most affected by AIDS.

But, as the epidemic progressed, the failures increasingly reflected our inability to strike a clear balance between the interests of society and the interests of individuals. In particular, we failed to use the proven tools possessed by the field of public health to fulfill what should be the first responsibility in an epidemic: the protection of the uninfected.

When I became Commissioner of Health in 1986, the Department of Health had counted some 7,000 cases of AIDS in the city. When I left my post at the end of the Koch administration in 1990, the number was 20,000; by 1992, it was up to 40,000 cases. By the middle of the decade, the number will be over 60,000.

If we know where it is going, and how it is transmitted, why can't we stop, or at least slow, this virus? That is the story of this book, which begins not with the epidemic's past, but with its current shape and future.

# The Shape of the Epidemic

My years as Health Commissioner were also the years in which the shape of the HIV epidemic became quite clear. More accurately, one should speak of the "shapes" of the epidemic, because of the different and sometimes oddly contrasting local and national patterns within this worldwide epidemic. Even within the United States, the patterns are diverse, which adds complexity to attempts to predict the epidemic's scope and future course.

In Africa, especially in a dozen countries of East and South Central Africa, AIDS has assumed cataclysmic proportions. In the most intensely infected urban (and some rural) areas, almost one-third of the entire adult population is currently infected. Transmission proceeds virtually unabated. Almost all infection is heterosexual and, by extension, from pregnant woman to fetus. Hundreds of thousands of small children are infected, and millions more will become "AIDS Orphans" as their parents die.

In contrast, in San Francisco, over 90 percent of AIDS cases in the first decade of the epidemic resulted from homosexual transmission. The impact of the epidemic, and the response to it, has been centered around the large and influential San Francisco gay community.

And yet again in contrast, in the blighted inner cities of northern New Jersey, most early cases resulted from the sharing of needles and syringes by drug addicts, and then transmission from addicts to sexual partners and their unborn children.

These oversimplified patterns conceal a more complex reality: the hypothetical concept of "pure epidemiologic patterns" is, of course, a very crude exaggeration, and is employed here only to make the point that homosexual, heterosexual, and injection-mediated (for example, by shared needles among drug addicts) transmission are the three primary factors determining the spread of the HIVirus: in any one given locality, the way in which these three factors are combined will produce the characteristic demographic pattern of AIDS for that locality.

In different locales, different mixes of the three primary factors predominate. Over time, as the epidemic proceeds, the mix of factors within a given locale will probably change. In New York, for example, the earliest recognized major factor of transmission was homosexual sex, though intense transmission among drug injectors was taking place at the same time. This gave New York a pattern of AIDS in the early years that was intermediate between—yet combined the characteristics of—San Francisco and northern New Jersey.

With the secondary flow of infection in the late 1980s to heterosexual partners of drug abusers (and to a much lesser extent, female partners of bisexual men), some parts of New York City began to acquire a pattern of HIV transmission resembling the pattern in Haiti, with mixed hetero- and homosexual transmission. In Haiti, however, the virus's major route of entry into the female population was probably via bisexual men, rather than via the drug abusers most responsible in the urban United States. Some observers fear the possibility of a shift in New York City in the 1990s to what came to be called "the African model" in which the epidemic would be maintained at high intensity by heterosexual activity not dependent on known contact with drug injectors.

In most other urban areas of the United States, including high-incidence cities such as Miami and the District of Columbia, the epidemic in the first decade was much like New York's, less intense perhaps, but still determined by infection among drug addicts (mostly male and in most cities heavily black and Hispanic) and their sex partners (mostly female and mostly minority), and among homosexual males (initially mostly white and middle class).

As the virus spread into secondary cities, suburban areas, and rural areas, the predominant mode of transmission was among homosexual men though, as in New York, a heavier infection of drug injectors and their heterosexual partners occurred than was generally realized. For example, black drug addicts in Atlanta disseminated the virus widely and heterosexually among poor rural blacks throughout the state of Georgia. But in general, the epidemic in small towns and rural areas was rather accurately perceived as an infection among gay men, a large proportion of whom were leading closeted lives.

The middle-class suburban and small-town nightmare of a coming "heterosexual breakout of the virus," the caricature of which was the bisexual tennis pro at the local country club, never came true—and most likely, never will. In reality, a low-intensity but persistent heterosexual spread of the virus was already occurring, but it was driven by drug users and heavily concentrated among poor and minority residents living in the shadows of wealthier neighbors.

## The Future of the Epidemic

Perhaps even more serious than the rising numbers of AIDS cases during my years as Health Commissioner was the shift in the epidemic's pathway. The late 1980s witnessed the great epidemiologic shift—away from white gay males and toward inner-city minority heterosexuals.

This is not to say that gay males will be free of AIDS. On the contrary, the mid-1990s in New York City will bear the full impact of AIDS illness and mortality among gay men. As the large majority of infected gay men who acquired the virus in the early 1980s become severely ill, and as the palliation of currently available treatment is exhausted, they will die. The highly visible impact of this flood of deaths will give the appearance of an increasing epidemic, which has in fact, at least among gay men, long since peaked.

Looking retrospectively at New York City, one can see that the number of new cases occurring annually among white gay men began to plateau perhaps as early as 1988, and by 1990 was probably actually declining. In part this was due to a reduction in risk behavior among gay men, but in part it was also due to a near-saturation of existing infection among those gay men whose individual behavior put them at highest risk. It is important to realize that the backlog of intense infection, and the long years of lag between infection and illness, provide the fuel for persistent illness and deaths among gay men. This will last (and continue to cumulate to very high numbers) throughout the 1990s. This is despite the leveling off of new cases of AIDS and a much-heralded earlier decline in new HIV transmission rates among gay men.

This, after all, is a very "smart" virus. While the human immunodeficiency virus is less transmissible than many other viruses (for example, those that cause hepatitis), and seems to require direct access to the bloodstream via injection or an abraded surface, once infection takes place the virus's evolutionary strategy is a highly successful one. Infection is clinically almost silent for a long period of time, but infectiousness to others persists. The virus enters the genetic material of infected cells—literally turning those cells into factories to produce more virus. Though the infection is, at present, invariably fatal, the infected individual lives for many years, an extremely efficient mechanism for the evolutionary success of the virus, which thus has every opportunity for survival and also infection of new individuals. This is a virus whose evolutionary strategy is designed for the long haul—in individuals and in populations.

Thus, though new infections among gay men in New York City have been leveling off or decreasing, the greatest impact of disease and then of death will not be apparent until years later, in the mid- and late-1990s.

No similar leveling off of new cases among New York's intravenous drug users was evident by 1990, and among women the rates of the appearance of new cases continue to increase, though women remained in absolute terms less than a quarter of all the persons with AIDS in the city.

The best current estimates are that the cumulative number of AIDS cases in New York City will reach 60,000 (about one-half of whom will be still alive) shortly after 1993—and that fully half of all those cases will have been first diagnosed since 1990! Among them, cases of women and infants, minorities, and drug users will be about 25 percent higher than was predicted by earlier estimates, and cases among gay men more than 40 percent lower than earlier estimates. The "average" person who was infected with HIV back in 1990 would not be expected to develop AIDS until around the turn of the century, or to die before 2002.

Those trends, of course, will be further accentuated if the additional 60,000 to 75,000 cases of HIV illness not yet diagnosed as AIDS are counted. Most of these will have been even more recently infected, and conform even more strongly to the clear trends in the epidemic, with increasing involvement of minority heterosexuals.

The likely course of the epidemic, in New York City and nationally, over the next decade, encompasses several fundamental points.

HIV illness will move more deeply into poor and minority communities, with the most striking feature being the broadening of heterosexual transmission and the gradual decline of the classical risk behaviors of male-to-male sex and intravenous drug use/needle sharing. These original two factors will remain important, but will no longer be in and of themselves adequate markers for the limits of risk in minority communities. Cases of AIDS in both men and especially in women will increasingly appear "spontaneously," with neither partner able to identify a link with drug injection or with a specific former sex partner. Thus, transmission of the virus will "dive below the surface" of our current markers of risk. As a consequence, a broader approach to AIDS education messages, counseling and testing for heterosexual populations living in high-risk areas, and the public health tracing and alerting of sexual partners of individuals known to be HIV-infected, will be increasingly important.

Though the HIVirus is transmitted less efficiently in penile-vaginal, as opposed to penile-rectal intercourse, the large reservoir of infection among minority heterosexuals will provide for ongoing transmission to secondary (and even further removed) partners of the man or woman originally infected through needle sharing, especially in neighborhoods with a high prevalence of other sexually transmitted diseases and very large numbers of partners related to sex-for-drugs prostitution.

By the end of the 1990s, HIV infection will be endemic (persistent but at a lessened level of intensity) in minority neighborhoods —much as syphilis was in the 1930s. In effect, a weaker reflection of the "African pattern" of AIDS will indeed hang over minority neighborhoods, albeit at a much lower level of intensity than in Africa, with the possibility of HIV infection shadowing heterosexual relationships, whether long-term or casual. It is difficult to predict how high the rates of infection will be, but it is not unreasonable to suppose that in the most affected poor minority neighborhoods, 10–15 percent of reproductive-age men and women will be infected. This, of course, will lead to the birth of a steady stream of HIV-infected infants and the orphaning of a steady stream of older, uninfected children as mothers and fathers die of AIDS. To get a sense of the magnitude of the AIDS Orphan problem: New York City will have 10,000–20,000 of these children by the late 1990s.

The relative inefficiency of heterosexual transmission will keep the chain reaction of HIV transmission from accelerating as explosively as it did among homosexual males, but there will be a sustained high level of new infections in minority communities at least through the first decade of the next century. Again, this is a "smart" virus, whose life cycle of infection is measured in more than a decade.

The resulting burden of illness and death will, of course, severely strain the social and medical systems of these communities upon which large proportions of their residents depend. In an especially cruel "Catch 22," the greater and more rapid the development of life-prolonging therapy for HIV illness, the more intense the crushing pressures on hospitals and health care systems in hard-pressed cities such as New York will be.

With regard to the gay community, the 1990s will witness three trends. The most visible will be the horrific toll of illness and death described above, as the many tens of thousands initially infected in the 1980s become seriously ill and eventually succumb. With current rates of existing infection at 25–30 percent or more among self-identified gay men in cities such as New York and San Francisco, the eventual cumulative effect of severe HIV illness and AIDS deaths among gay men will be staggering.

Second, additional gay and bisexual men will continue to be infected with HIV at a persistent but lower rate than currently is the case. The behavioral changes of the 1980s toward safer sex practices are not being maintained with anything like their initial success. And the infection is moving from its big city base into smaller cities and communities that lack strongly organized, visible, and vocal gay communities. Indeed, evidence emerged in the late 1980s of a resurgence of risky behavior among many gays and of a sizable proportion of homosexual and bisexual men who had never changed their behavior.

In the understandable enthusiasm about the achievements of "safer sex education" among gay men in the mid-1980s, often lost sight of was the fact that most of the documented gains were statistical and far from absolute. For example, a reduction in average numbers of sex partners from fifty to twenty, or a proportion of men engaging in receptive anal intercourse decreasing from 15 percent to 8 percent, or $x$ percent of men stating that they used condoms $y$ percent of the time. This is not unlike playing Russian roulette only half as often but with twice as many bullets in the revolver. In fact, as the percentage of infected gay men in a given community rose, the actual risk of infection to an individual also rose, even though he may have actually had a smaller number of partners.

The large reservoir of infection among sexually active gay men, combined with the long time lag between infection and illness, will continually create new infections and maintain a high enough level of transmission to keep the cycle turning.

This will lead to the third trend: a high level of endemic infection and illness that will persist among homosexual and bisexual men, generating a less dramatic caseload than before, but posing a prevention and treatment dilemma that will endure for decades. Well into the twenty-first century, HIV infection will remain the first item on the list of possible diagnoses that will spring to the mind of a physician examining a gay man with a chronic disease. One of the characteristics that makes epidemiologists call this virus smart is its ability to survive. It will endure for a long time to come.

Beyond the sustained endemic levels among minorities and homosexual men, AIDS among white and middle-class New York heterosexuals will remain at low levels, though the absolute number of cases will increase—both those that are directly traceable to bisexual and drug-using partners, and those that are one or several heterosexual partners removed from identifiable risk factors. HIV illness will not be a very rare diagnosis among middle-class heterosexuals, but neither will it be very frequent. It is likely that, by the mid-1990s, the middle-class perception of the direct threat posed by the epidemic may return to feelings of a personal insulation from risk of infection. This may lead to indifference to those with greater risk—a situation similar to that of the early 1980s, before the "heterosexual panic" brought AIDS awareness to the middle class.

In other major urban centers with significant poor/minority and gay populations, the evolution of the epidemic will be similar to that described for New York City, with varying levels of intensity and varying time lags. The most important variables will be, as before, the size of the homosexual community and the rates of drug addiction (particularly as associated with shooting galleries) within a given city. In cities where the drug epidemic—especially of crack cocaine—is currently being "imported," cases of HIV infection are also being imported, via infected drug dealers coming from more drug- and HIV-established centers, and able to infect new customers and sexual partners.

In smaller towns and rural areas, the epidemic's focused predilection for homosexuals as well as heterosexuals belonging to poor/minority groups will, if anything, be even more marked than in the major cities. Though the incidence of AIDS will increase steadily in rural America in the 1990s, it will be largely mediated by the now familiar two factors: male-to-male sex and drug abuse. Thus the large majority of rural Americans infected will be poor, minority heterosexuals or homosexual men. A particular feature of HIV transmission in small towns and rural areas will involve the spread of the virus among gay men leading closeted lives, and the transmission to women from closeted bisexual partners.

There is no way to head off this facet of the epidemic without widespread and vigorous use of the antibody test, mandatory public health reporting of infection, and contact tracing and notification of partners of infected individuals.

Occasional explosive local outbreaks of HIV illness will occur in impoverished rural communities with high levels of substance abuse and sexually transmitted diseases, such as have already occurred in Belle Glade, Florida, and in rural Georgia. There will also be rare and sporadic-seeming occurrences of cases among the rural middle class.

Thus, the future of the HIV epidemic in the United States will be as follows: many more cases, far more widespread around the country, but still focused and concentrated in the major urban centers; a much larger proportion of transmission will be heterosexual, but most of this will occur in poor and minority communities where drug abuse and high levels of other sexually transmitted diseases drive the virus onward.

The "heterosexual breakout," so feared in the mid-1980s by the white middle class, has, in fact, already occurred in major cities, and is poised for expansion to the rest of the country. But like most public health tragedies, it predominantly afflicts the poor and the disadvantaged, and will continue to do so. The relatively uncommon case of the Park Avenue socialite infected by a bisexual former boyfriend, which receives such media attention, is multiplied several thousandfold among her black and Hispanic counterparts, who receive considerably less public concern and who, being at much higher risk, deserve far more intensive health protection.

I have learned from frustrating experience that what I have written here will be condemned by some as racist or homophobic. It is neither, but rather a sober prediction of the probable future of the HIVirus in this country. This is what is going to happen, and this should allow us to prepare more carefully for the likely consequences of coming developments: what social, economic, and other consequences might follow, how wild card events or occurrences might modify the future, and what measures must be taken to try to stem the future ravages of the epidemic.

The most immediate consequence of the epidemic's probable future track is that public attitudes will very likely shift back again to the alienated us/them perceptions of the early 1980s. As middle-class society, especially outside the big cities, begins to view the HIVirus as posing little personal threat of infection, society may react with both (1) increasing discrimination against homosexuals and minorities seen as vulnerable to AIDS, and (2) increasing political reluctance to support public funding for research, treatment, and other needed services. This would be a great tragedy, not only because of the inequities it creates, but also because the economic and social effects of the epidemic will place major burdens on the entire country. Enlightened self-interest demands that the entire population commit to combating the epidemic.

To encourage middle-class response to the epidemic's challenge requires first, reinforced education about the nature of the epidemic and its personal risks; second, a clear understanding of the epidemic's widespread social and economic costs; and, third—and the most neglected to date—that affected groups must place their own best efforts behind effective methods of prevention, acting beyond narrow perceptions of self-interest.

The gay community, which did such a spectacular early job of educating itself and others about risk reduction, and of developing volunteer services, uniformly resisted public health proposals for active prevention measures, such as widespread antibody testing, mandatory reporting of infection to public health authorities, and vigorous contact tracing of the partners of infected people. Gay opposition has been based on political self-interest and on genuine fears of government repression of homosexuals. Just how damaging such self-interest can be—to the group as well as the general public —can be seen in the controversy over use of the antibody test to protect the blood supply.

Well before the discovery of the HIVirus, it became clear that AIDS could be transmitted through infected blood transfusions. Blood bank officials were in a difficult position. They were pressured by gay leaders not to "stigmatize" homosexuals by publicly discouraging gays from donating blood. Blood banks feared a loss of blood donations and resultant shortages of critically needed blood supplies if the public lost confidence in the system. Valuable time was lost as officials wrestled with the development of procedures that would safeguard the blood supply to the extent possible, but would also avoid what was unfortunately interpreted by blood bank directors as "undue public concern" (this was, of course, long before the HIV antibody test made assurance of safety of donated units practicable).

Throughout 1982, national representatives of the blood banks were assuring the public that "there is no evidence that there is the danger of AIDS transmission through the blood supply." Thus, with the use of those words "there is no evidence," the impression was once again given (as it was in New York with regard to heterosexual transmission) that no risk existed when, in fact, the truth was quite the opposite.

Protection of the blood supply was the first area in which prevention efforts became critical. In the absence of a test to screen out infected units of donated blood, the New York Blood Center and other major blood banks around the country quietly adopted, in 1983, a policy known as "self-exclusion." Individuals (primarily homosexual men) who thought they might be at risk of HIV infection were asked not to donate blood, and cooperation with gay organizations and leaders was sought to quietly "pass the word" not to donate blood. It is, of course, impossible to know how effective this policy proved.

Payments to individuals for blood donations to be used for transfusion had long been illegal in New York State, and commercial blood banks were not a factor in the transfusion picture. Had this not been so, and with so many infected drug addicts who would have presumably been selling their blood, the city's blood supply might have undergone large-scale and ongoing infection. Also, though this was little known, the New York Blood Center received a large amount of its transfusion blood from Europe, principally from Switzerland, and in retrospect this too was an added safety element.

Nevertheless, by the end of 1990, over a hundred New Yorkers were known to have acquired AIDS via infected blood transfusions. These infections were virtually all acquired before the HIV antibody test was available to screen donations. However, the true number of transfusion-infected New Yorkers must have been far higher, in the several hundreds, because (1) not all those people infected before 1985 would have developed AIDS by 1990 and (2) according to New York Blood Center figures, almost 60 percent of all people who receive a blood transfusion die within a year, not from the effects of the transfusion, but from the serious medical and surgical conditions that caused them to need the transfusion in the first place. These numbers, of course, must be placed in the perspective of the millions of units of blood transfused annually in the New York region, blood that in many cases is urgently needed to maintain life.

Exclusion of blood donations on a self-stated behavioral basis should have been more vigorous (for example, a confidential questionnaire asking about sexual preference and drug use should have been part of the donation process beginning in 1982, with the exclusion of all donors who indicated any risk behavior). In addition, surgeons and internists should have exercised far more judicious decisions as to when transfusion was medically imperative. Beyond these two reforms, very little more could have been done to protect the blood supply until the antibody test became available. Blood bank officials lived in constant dread that public confidence in the laboriously constructed system of free and anonymous blood donation would be destroyed, and theirs was a reasonable dilemma. Each time a publicized event concerning AIDS and the blood supply occurred, donations dropped; the public would not accept that AIDS could not be contracted from donating, as opposed to receiving, blood, and a prevalent, though incorrect, attitude was that it was best to just avoid any and all contact with the system.

In this context, the arrival of a reliable antibody test was of the greatest benefit. However, when the test became available in spring 1985, many voices sought to limit its use, because of fear that the test would be used to stigmatize or discriminate against people found to be infected. Fortunately, the federal Food and Drug Administration proceeded to license the test, and states made it widely available for screening of the blood supply. Had this not happened by the late 1980s, a disastrous increase in transfusion-mediated HIV infection would surely have occurred, and an equally disastrous collapse of the blood banking system would have followed.

The availability, reliability, and widespread use of the HIV antibody test for the screening and protection of the blood supply was a technical achievement of the highest order. Blood banks rapidly developed large-scale systems of screening, with subsequent exclusion of units found to be infected, and confidential notification of those donors of the infected units. However, there was no referral for public health follow-up of infected individuals, which could have been the basis of a contact tracing mechanism that would have averted many further HIV infections in those early years.

It is widely suspected among health personnel that the blood banking system keeps a cross-referenced index of donors who have been shown to be HIV infected, and that the information is shared among blood banks—but not, of course, passed on to local public health authorities. If indeed this is true, and I believe that it is, there is no indication that this information has been used in a discriminatory fashion, shared with health insurers, or that the confidentiality of the system has been breached. In my view, such a system-wide list of infected donors is a legitimate use of HIV antibody test information, and would have further appropriate and significant benefits if linked to confidential public health reporting and partner notification systems.

The blood screening system, though highly reliable, was not absolutely foolproof. As early as 1987, a documented case (from Colorado) was reported in which a transfusion recipient acquired HIV infection from a unit of blood donated by a person during the "window period" after infection but before antibodies to the virus could be detected. This rare but predictable event, reported by the federal Centers for Disease Control, provoked another round of severe public anxiety about the blood supply. There were calls for "testing everyone" who had received a blood transfusion since the introduction of the antibody test in 1985. The position of most public health officials, including myself, was that this would be excessive. Rather, it made sense to understand that a spectrum of risk existed, ranging from very low in someone who had received a single unit of blood in New York since 1985, to very high in someone who had received multiple transfusions in 1982 and 1983. Those who were concerned about having received transfusions since 1977 were advised to consult their physicians about the desirability of being tested for HIV infection.

Further, the blood banks and hospitals worked together to construct a "look-back" system, to identify units of blood during and after 1985 that may have come from persons who were later diagnosed with AIDS. The hospitals would then notify the physicians of individuals who had received potentially dangerous units, and the physicians would notify the individuals. Many physicians were quite reluctant to participate in this process, for fear of legal liability. In any event, no post-1985 infections caused by transfusion in New York City were identified.

A distressing sidelight to the blood donation screening issue had to do with the possibilities of transmitting HIV infection through other means of "donated" tissues: bone marrow and organ transplants, and most commonly, artificial insemination. The Department of Health was aware in New York City of sizable numbers of women undergoing artificial insemination to become pregnant, and of certain physicians who maintained sperm banks with commercial semen donors, a significant proportion of whom were thought to be homosexuals. By late 1986 we were urging the State Health Department to require that all donated and transplanted tissues and organs, including semen especially, involve a mandated current HIV test of the donor. In 1987 and 1988 the Centers for Disease Control reported a series of HIV infections acquired via transplanted tissues. It also became clear that HIV infection could be (though rarely) transmitted through breast milk, and there were no protective regulations governing human milk banks.

The state's pace on developing and enacting these regulations was glacial. In 1987 and 1988 one of our departmental research projects concerning artificial insemination yielded alarming results. We were studying a group of women who had been inseminated through the sperm bank of a physician with a large private practice. Of his first thirty patients who agreed to be tested, two (who had no other risk factors) turned out to be HIV positive. We determined that they most probably had been infected via the insemination. The physician was reluctant to "call back" all of his inseminated patients to alert them to their risk and to urge them to be tested. It was only when we applied direct threats of public exposure and whatever legal sanctions we could conceive of under the "hazard to public health" category of the Health Code, that he cooperated. With our assistance and pressure, he eventually reached all 123 of his insemination patients. Most were tested, and several were found to be infected.

This tragic episode added impetus to our calls for the state to implement regulations for mandatory HIV testing of organ and sperm donors. Not until early 1989 were such regulations enacted. Undoubtedly additional women were HIV-infected during this time; it is possible that a number of their offspring (from the inseminated or even from a subsequent pregnancy) have died of AIDS. Most of these women, of course, have not yet developed symptoms of HIV illness, and most have no idea that they are infected, and are infectious to others. This is another example of the consequences of our failure to use the HIV antibody test to its maximum advantage, certainly to protect all individuals receiving sperm or tissue from another individual, and more generally among all women contemplating or entering pregnancy.

The appearance of the HIV antibody test was accompanied by much controversy. Since only wide-scale experience with the test could demonstrate its accuracy, part of the concern was based on the fear of significant numbers of results that would be false-positive (indicating HIV infection in someone who is actually free of infection) and false-negative (a test indicating the absence of infection in someone who is actually infected with HIV). But much more vocal were the fears of the gay community that the test would be applied in a mandatory fashion to persons considered to be at risk, and that it would be used to discriminate not only against individuals actually infected with the virus, but in some way against all homosexuals.

In practice, when used under standard conditions, the HIV antibody test proved to be among the most accurate and useful diagnostic entities we possess. Its predictive value significantly outperforms most laboratory and diagnostic techniques routinely employed and accepted today throughout various fields of medicine.

In New York, the AIDS advocates' view of the antibody test as a danger rather than an opportunity, and their framing of the arguments concerning testing as a civil libertarian rather than a public health issue, were quickly accepted, without significant or vigorous debate. Rather than seeking the maximum utility of the test while guarding against its abuse, the context became one of always restricting its use unless and until a very tight cocoon of safeguards against abuse could be wrapped around it.

Thus, in most jurisdictions, and certainly in New York, antibody testing was always to be voluntary, never mandatory, always to be preceded by rather elaborate "pretest counseling" that emphasized to the potential "testee" all the dangers and possible discriminatory consequences of the test results. Testing itself was to be performed in an anonymous setting (solely in an anonymous setting if publicly funded), where the counselor and laboratory did not know the identity of the person being tested. When the test was performed by a private physician, the sample was to be sent, coded, to the public health laboratory (the city and state public health labs were, until late 1988, the only laboratories in New York permitted to perform the procedure, except for blood banks performing donation screening), and the public health agencies would never know the identity behind the samples. Elaborate and specific written consent had to be obtained by the physician, who also had to certify that, in addition to pretest counseling, "post-test counseling" would be provided to both HIV-positive and HIV-negative patients.

None of these measures were in themselves bad, and it was certainly important to protect the rights and confidentiality of patients against unwanted or misunderstood testing and against discrimination flowing from breached confidentiality of test results. But the zeal with which these protective efforts became civil libertarian dogma, the lengths to which the details of counseling and testing regulations were pursued, the fear that surrounded the test—all these inhibited the growth of testing, and made its use in appropriate medical circumstances more difficult.

For example, by the late 1980s the medical importance of women knowing their HIV status when they considered pregnancy or were in early prenatal care was undeniable. Yet instead of devising ways to expand the routine—but voluntary—use of antibody testing, sustained and powerful efforts restricted its use. These misguided efforts seemed to be intended, in some bizarre way, either to "protect" women by withholding the information from them, or to "protect" them from possible discrimination should they be tested and the results be disclosed to others. In dismal fact, these efforts only ensured the restriction to a very small proportion of women at risk within such inner cities as New York, Los Angeles, Miami, and Washington, D.C. of the information that was of major, if not critical, implication for their health and that of the children they were bearing.

The eight city-funded anonymous test sites we created in New York City provided a critical service, but it was clear as early as 1987 that the need was for vastly expanded counseling and testing services, available at every point of clinical contact: the doctor's office, the clinic or hospital, the family planning or abortion clinic. Most testing in New York was actually being done confidentially and in clinical settings rather than at the anonymous test sites. The many restrictions around testing, wherever performed, prevented appropriate growth. In particular, physicians found the test requirements burdensome, and the state made little effort to streamline the process.

I strongly and repeatedly supported the commercial laboratories' request to State Health Commissioner David Axelrod that a limited number of private laboratories be permitted to perform the first stage of the test directly for physicians, with the confirmatory second-stage test on positive specimens to be done by our own city or state laboratories. This would have opened up testing to thousands of additional physicians, who felt themselves unable to deal with the cumbersome system of sending their specimens, along with coded information and informed consent attestations, to city and state labs. Doctors were used to having commercial laboratories pick up specimens at their offices in the afternoon and return results in the shortest possible interval, often the next morning. As it was, with sustained effort and much tablepounding, I was only able to get our own city laboratory turnaround time of coded test results back to physicians on a ten-day basis, and I knew that the commercial labs would be able to do much better. In 1988, only 5 percent of the 25,000 physicians practicing in New York City had ever submitted an HIV antibody test specimen to the Department of Health. Allowing the commercial sector to come in and perform the laboratory analysis of specimens would have multiplied that manyfold, and rapidly.

Dr. Axelrod refused to allow any commercial laboratories to do HIV testing, citing vague grounds of "quality control" and "confidentiality" problems. We argued in vain that a limited number of the larger, higher quality labs could be closely monitored in the process, but Axelrod remained inflexible. Finally, in 1988, the State Health Department agreed to allow New York City teaching hospitals to apply for permits to perform HIV antibody tests on-site; we quickly certified eighteen hospitals around the city to do just that, and the volume of clinically based testing rose significantly.

But the bells and whistles of the regulations surrounding testing, and the attitudes labeling it an infringement on civil rights rather than a tool for public health protection were widespread (not least within my own department staff). Creative and vigorous use of the test never took off. In my view, the failure to use the antibody test to its maximum, while carefully guarding against its abuse, will be seen in the future as one of the major and most important missed opportunities of the epidemic.

The gay community was not the only community to define the epidemic socially and politically rather than medically. Minority communities have largely ignored the HIV threat and the need for aggressive preventive efforts to protect themselves, and particularly their female members. Both gay and minority communities would gain both practical and symbolic advantages by reversing their current stands.

The demographic and social consequences of the AIDS epidemic in the 1990s will be enormous. Without question, the size and characteristics of gay male communities, especially in magnet cities such as New York and San Francisco, will be fundamentally altered. No population can experience a mortality among its members of 25–30 percent, even spread over a decade and a half, without being altered and marked by the experience. Consider that the loss of life in the Soviet Union in the Second World War was approximately 5 percent of the population, and you may have some idea of what the AIDS epidemic will mean to the gay community (or, for that matter, to the hardest hit African nations).

It is likely that the character of entire neighborhoods, such as New York's Greenwich Village, will be devastated; the social and professional character of the city will shift to new, and as yet unguessed, patterns. The artistic, cultural, and fashion enterprises which are particularly important to New York's world standing and economy have traditionally included large numbers of gay men. By the mid-1990s, the toll of the epidemic will have made such large inroads into these fields as to alter them visibly.

Like its predecessor major plagues, AIDS will wreak a havoc similar to the devastation of war, especially among homosexual men living in concentrated communities. The tragedy of death among the young is, of course, far from uncommon. But the repeated and wholesale loss of friends and neighbors, surrounded by a community whose members know that a large proportion of themselves will also fall victim to a particularly painful and gruesome death, has a far larger impact.

This has been a reality for gay men since the mid-1980s. But as the numbers of deaths rise, reaching into the tens of thousands per year in New York City in the mid-1990s, the consequences will be greater still. Significant numbers of gay men will flee the most heavily affected cities, especially as the death tolls mount; this trend has already been documented, especially from San Francisco to the rural Western states. Many of these men are already infected. Many will live closeted lives in more conservative communities, some adopting bisexual identities. The potential of further penetration of the epidemic into currently less affected areas is obvious.

The impact of AIDS on minority communities will be less sharply focused, but probably heavier. The peak of illness and deaths among black and Hispanic New Yorkers will occur somewhat later than among gay men, in the second half of the 1990s, and will be spread out over a longer period.

But the effects of the epidemic are already evident in infant and adult mortality rates, and in the recurrence of other infectious diseases, such as tuberculosis, among poor and minority populations. In 1992, nationwide public fear was aroused by the recognition that tuberculosis was rapidly rising, especially in the inner cities. Of greatest concern was the increasing identification of strains of tuberculosis that were resistant to several of the antibiotics commonly used in treatment. But the increase in tuberculosis had been going on in these cities, including New York, for almost a decade. New York city epidemiologists had shown that up to one-third of the tuberculosis increase in the mid-1980s had been among adult men who were immuno-compromised by HIV. Not only were and are HIV-infected people most at risk of becoming ill with tuberculosis under these circumstances, but they also serve as a potential reservoir for the infection of others, including health workers and others who come into prolonged and close contact with them. Though otherwise healthy people exposed to the tuberculosis organism are not very likely to become ill with tuberculosis, a small fraction indeed will, and the prospect of this widespread risk of infection with multiply-resistant tuberculosis organisms is a public health nightmare that must be taken with the utmost seriousness. In one sense, it is an only slightly diminished version of the worst nightmare of AIDS: that the illness would become transmissible from person to person by more casual contact. In this case, it is drug-resistant tuberculosis that can be spread, initially by HIV-infected individuals, to any close contact in the population.

AIDS will cut a broad swath through the health gains that have been made in the past twenty years among the disadvantaged, and will reverse progress on key health indicators. It will overwhelm attempts to provide adequate social services: welfare, housing, child protection, foster care, and mental health services, in the hardest hit cities. In what is perhaps its most insidious effect, AIDS will likely cripple the possibilities of reconstructing the base of the black inner-city family for the next two decades or more.

There will be severe effects on the general economy of New York, probably peaking in the late 1990s. In direct terms, the strains on health and social services will be substantial. The estimated $7 billion (25 percent contributed by the city) needed for meeting only the direct costs of the epidemic between 1990 and 1993 will strain the city's budget. The other side of this Hobbesian choice is, of course, the social disruption and associated costs to be borne if services fall significantly short of what is needed, as they have to date. The increased burden of illness during the mid-1990s will mean that associated costs will continue to increase, and probably for some time afterward, say until the early years of the next century.

There are wild card events that could, by their occurrence, sharply change the course or impact of the epidemic. Most of them have very little chance of actually occurring, but all of them are frequently speculated upon, and most of them are exaggerations of less dramatic developments that, though much less stark, do have a realistic chance of appearing.

The first wild card—one put forward by many as a doomsday scenario—would be a sudden change in the nature of the HIVirus itself, or the appearance of a new strain, a sort of Super-HIV that would be much more easily communicable or much more lethal.

The probability of this occurring in its purest sense is almost nil. Though the HIVirus is one that mutates rapidly, like the influenza virus, and though we already know of two major distinct strains (HIV-1, responsible for most of the epidemic in the United States, and HIV-2, a less virulent strain found principally in West Africa), it would be extremely unlikely for a sudden mutation to produce an HIV strain that was transmissible by casual contact, or that ran to its full expression of disease and death of the host within weeks or months. The evolutionary niche carved out by HIV for itself is one in which slow but sure spread, lifelong infection, and prolonged survival of the infected host are advantageous to the virus. In its evolutionary strategy, the HIVirus is more a marathon runner than a sprinter. The future major patterns of HIV infection are virtually certain to remain within traditional boundaries. The major, and likely, exception to this is the type of scenario outlined above for tuberculosis, where the HIV-infected population becomes a reservoir for some other infection to which the general, non HIV-infected population is then exposed.

A more likely—in fact almost certain—danger is that as antiviral therapy expands, resistant strains of HIV will emerge. Indeed laboratory and clinical evidence of the development of HIV resistance to the antiviral drug AZT already exists.

It is the associated infections with other viruses, bacteria, and fungi that directly cause a large proportion of the symptoms of disease in people with HIV illness. These are the so-called "opportunistic infections" (opportunistic because they take advantage of the depleted immune defense system of the HIV-infected person). It is to be expected that drug resistance among the opportunistic infections (particularly those that are viral or bacterial in nature) will increase, and that those opportunistic infections which are most successfully treated will themselves be replaced by others increasingly difficult to treat. This phenomenon of successful therapy begetting the next generation of therapeutic dilemmas (what Rene Dubos called "the mirage of health") is the virtually universal experience with antibiotic therapy. There is no reason to expect that it will be any different with the HIVirus. There will be no magic bullet solution to the treatment of AIDS, though we can confidently expect therapy to become far more powerful and for patients to survive far longer than is currently the case.

But HIV infection will remain a difficult, time consuming, expensive, and problematic illness to treat, even under the most optimistic scenarios. The persistence and power of this virus, and the difficulty and costs of treatment, make vigorous and effective prevention of transmission an urgent issue.

Much improved antiviral therapy is almost certain to emerge during the 1990s, with the appearance of progressively effective agents that act against various stages of the life cycle of HIV: preventing the virus from entering cells, inhibiting its replication within the cell, blocking the release of virus from infected cells, etc.

AIDS will take on the character of a treatable but not curable chronic disease by the mid- or late-1990s. This will spell hope, longer survival, and a much heightened quality of life for millions of infected people.

A less hopeful corollary of this is that therapy for HIV illness will remain complex, not truly curative, and very costly. The faster therapeutic knowledge grows, the greater the demands will be upon health care systems in cities such as New York, as larger numbers of patients, surviving for longer periods of time, require greater amounts of increasingly complex and expensive hospital and outpatient services. And as the proportion and numbers of AIDS patients who depend on publicly funded health care grow, the pressures on the public sector will grow, and the current decay of the public hospital system accelerates.

The second wild card would be the development of a vaccine providing effective primary prevention. The most optimistic researchers place the earliest possible date of a widely available vaccine in the late-1990s, and many are pessimistic about developing an effective vaccine at all in the foreseeable future. In any case, the testing of a vaccine for safety and efficacy poses especially difficult problems in the case of HIV, and would consume at least several years.

A vaccine is not at all likely to be available during the balance of the critical years of the U.S. epidemic—between now and 2000. Unless a supremely unlikely wild card is turned up, a vaccine will come too late to provide much of a major barrier to the growth of the epidemic itself in the United States.

Other forms of primary prevention, however, range from public health measures (behavioral change through education, public health reporting of infected people and tracing their contacts) to the probabilities of pharmacologic blocking of transmission (such as with penicillin for syphilis or drugs against tuberculosis). A chemical agent that can interrupt transmission is not a wild card, but likely to become a reality. One can predict that within the next few years it will be shown that one or more of the antiviral agents reduces infectiousness. That demonstration, of course, will end once and for all the debate as to the utility of the use of public health measures for the early identification of infected persons. It will become clear, as it should have several years earlier, that a primary objective that must be achieved is the early identification of the infected, and of those at high individual risk of infection.

Might there be a wild card shift or breakthrough in our knowledge about HIV? This has generally taken the shape of theories that "HIV is not the cause of AIDS" or that other cofactors are necessary for the progression to immune deficiency.

Disproving a negative is always difficult, but my view is that it is extremely unlikely that any discovery will negate or fundamentally change the existing view of the natural history of HIV infection. Current knowledge will be improved and modified, but it is highly improbable that we will suddenly find that we have been progressing down a blind alley, or even a wrong street.

The projection of the future epidemic in New York and in the rest of the nation outlined above is grim, even discounting the highly improbable wild card scenarios. It paints a picture of an epidemic that, from a long head start, has continued to outdistance worldwide efforts in prevention and treatment. AIDS will reach peak intensity of illness and death in the mid- and late-1990s, and then will simmer on at lower levels for several decades, mostly affecting homosexual men, drug abusers, and heterosexuals of minority and poverty groups. The entire society will pay a heavy price, in erosion of health and social services systems and general economic hemorrhage.

The major determinants of this scenario are already firmly in motion, and there is little prospect of reversing them. The major battles to stop the epidemic in its tracks were lost long ago: first, before we even knew the threat existed, and then, when we vacillated without taking strong and effective preventive action.

But we are not powerless against this virus. Though we may no longer be able to avert its major lines of advance, we do have the capacity to prevent transmission to many additional thousands, perhaps hundreds of thousands, of uninfected individuals. This is especially true in the case of minority citizens.

Those likely remedies which we can apply include education and behavioral change, the application of therapy (which has a dual role of probably reducing infectiousness and of increasing motivation for antibody testing), and the determined application of sound public health principles of prevention.

Concepts of public health are abstractions unless they lead to the improvement of health for many individuals. We have the capacity, even at this late hour in the epidemic, to use our increasing knowledge to save tens of thousands of lives, and to reduce by a corresponding amount the despair and social costs of the epidemic.

This is where we are today and where we're going. This book suggests how we got here and what we might have done differently —and should do differently in the future—to avert unnecessary suffering and death.

# 2

## The Stony Roads to Prevention and Treatment: What We Need To Do Now

THE TWIN OBJECTIVES IN AN EPIDEMIC ARE TO PROTECT THE UNINFECTED and to treat the sick.

Meeting these objectives in the face of the AIDS epidemic requires:

—vigorous public health actions that will limit the further spread of the HIVirus

—increased knowledge about the virus, in both biologic and social domains

—expanded access to needed health and social services for those who are HIV-infected

There are also many important secondary objectives in combating the epidemic, such as avoiding discrimination against those at greatest risk. These other objectives, however important, are just that: secondary objectives. They can be achieved. But we should not subordinate the primary objectives to them, as we have too often done in this epidemic.

The most urgent task is to fight the epidemic by reducing further transmission of the virus. We can do this, and do it while adhering to the civil rights and individual liberties of all those involved. But we should not, in response to the political agenda of any special interest or advocacy groups, avoid taking those actions that are necessary to protect the uninfected. Protecting the uninfected is the first duty. AIDS constitutes a public health emergency which carries within it extraordinary civil liberties issues. It does not constitute a civil liberties emergency which carries within it extraordinary public health issues. To date, we have not adequately understood that distinction.

For a considerable time after AIDS was recognized as an epidemic, neither preventing transmission nor treating the sick could be pursued through any specific measures. There was no known treatment for the infected, and there was no known method of diagnosing infected but not-ill people. Neither was there any medical means of preventing transmission of the virus from one person to another.

As it became clearer that AIDS was indeed caused by a virus transmissible through blood-to-blood or sexual contact but not through airborne or casual spread, hopes turned to limiting the scope of the epidemic through prevention. Until roughly 1987, five years after recognition of the epidemic, there was still no specific treatment against the virus and little evidence that any medical measures either prolonged life or decreased suffering.

Prevention could be focused either upon reducing the individual's risk of infection, or upon broader social measures to protect groups and communities as a whole. One approach, of course, does not exclude the other. In fact, the most effective preventive strategy would have been to combine both approaches in joint personal and community prevention. Unfortunately, the political context of AIDS tended to set personal and community perspectives off as opposing views, and to falsely identify attempts at traditional public health approaches as threats to civil liberties.

Research was focused on a direct attack on the HIVirus, or on drugs that would treat the opportunistic infections that took advantage of the depressed immune system. (A third possibility, rebuilding or "boosting" the immune system, seemed a less effective route to follow in the face of continued viral infection, and did not play a major early role in research or therapy.)

The pace of progress that occurred in treatment research (anti-HIVirus, or anti-opportunistic infections) is all the more remarkable because we were dealing, in both instances, with microorganisms against which no effective antibiotic therapy was available for standard application, and against which no treatment barrier to transmission was known when the epidemic began.

# Prevention

It is when we come to the policies of AIDS prevention, or perhaps one might better say the politics of AIDS prevention, that the greatest disagreements and the most bitter disputes have occurred. From my own perspective, as a public health physician, it is clear that policymakers have allowed narrow political and social considerations to override scientific ones, to the ultimate detriment of both.

However the accuracy of that is judged, what is certain is that the 1990s bring us to a new context of the epidemic, with new opportunities and new dangers.

The profiles of new infection, and the probabilities of further spread, are now focused in two settings. In the most affected urban areas, infection and future illness seriously threaten heterosexual minority residents in poor neighborhoods. Though drug use and the sexual behaviors associated with crack were important for heterosexual transmission, these communities will increasingly see the heterosexual spread of infection to secondary partners—that is, where no direct connection to drug use is obvious. Thus, the warning signals that have been the basis for much of AIDS prevention and education will be less and less relevant to the prevention of further spread. This has the utmost implication for the risks of adolescents, young women, and unborn infants in these poor and minority communities.

Elsewhere, in the less affected cities, smaller towns, suburbs, and rural areas, AIDS will remain more heavily clustered among gay and bisexual men and intravenous (IV) drug users. Small but constant seepage of infection to the female sexual partners of drug injectors and bisexuals will occur. Here again, the ability to reach closeted gay men and unsuspecting women at risk will be much more limited than was the case in the most affected urban areas in the 1980s.

In both settings, effective AIDS education and early case finding and partner notification must be applied urgently. Escalating effectiveness of early treatment of HIV infection adds to this urgency. Early identification of infection, and the availability of sharply expanded access to care now is clearly in the best interests of the individual as well as of society as a whole.

Though the hour is late, prevention is still the only way to make an impact on the overall epidemic. Prevention of further transmission can still spare the less infected communities from allowing the virus to get a solid foothold. Prevention can still mitigate the havoc that the virus is sure to cause in the high-prevalence cities, and save many thousands of lives.

On the prevention side, education and media campaigns that came to be labeled "risk reduction" were much less costly than drug development and testing and gave the impression of progress. However, it is far from certain that the mass media messages and individual counseling about behavior change had much of an effect in reducing actual rates of transmission of the virus, especially among drug injectors.

The largest proportion of infection among gay men and IV drug users had in fact taken place before the middle of the 1980s decade, long before the major prevention campaigns were in place. The much publicized decrease in transmission among gay men in San Francisco and New York, inferred from a sharp drop in the occurrence of oral and rectal gonorrhea and in syphilis among gay men, is much more likely to represent, rather than a response to governmental public health programs, the combination of two factors: word-of-mouth communication among gay men concerning ways to avoid infection and early efforts by private gay advocacy groups to spread those messages. Moreover, among both gay men and IV drug users, it is very likely that groups at highest risk, such as shooting gallery addicts and gay men with large numbers of sexual partners, were already so heavily saturated with infection that only lower-risk individuals were left uninfected and open to "prevention."

No persuasive evidence yet exists that either the mass media campaigns or the individual counseling associated with antibody testing have had a marked and sustained effect on sexual or drug abusing behavior, and thus on actually reducing transmission of the HIVirus sufficiently to lessen the speed or scope of the epidemic.

This is not to say that education and counseling are unimportant or ineffective. Undoubtedly, many individuals have altered their behaviors to prevent their own infection or that of others. But what is problematic is that this has occurred on a large enough scale to make a difference in the dynamics of the epidemic. Indeed, little evidence exists that this has happened with IV drug users, especially with regard to sexual behavior.

Which prevention strategies work and will alter the spread of AIDS poses a momentous question for the second decade of the epidemic, as the virus moves more deeply into inner-city heterosexual populations and spreads more widely among homosexuals and drug users in smaller towns and rural areas. Its answer is the key to the actual prevention opportunities that still lie before us, as opposed to the illusion of prevention that marked the early years of the epidemic.

Progress in both prevention and treatment of HIV infection depends upon understanding the basic biology, the natural history, and the social concomitants of the virus. At the beginning of the epidemic we were in effect starting from ground zero, uncertain even about whether this was an infectious process, or what the specific disease-causing agent might be.

As knowledge about the biology of the HIVirus crystallized, followed closely by a basic understanding of the natural history of the infection, understanding of the social and behavioral aspects of the epidemic lagged far behind.

Would political factors have been so powerful in determining the course public policy was to take if understanding of the biological basis of HIV infection had coincided with the epidemic? My own belief is that had the biology been better understood in the first few years, traditional public health prevention activities, such as reporting of infected individuals to public health departments and tracing sex and drug partners of those infected, would have been stronger. The social and political forces driving the response to the epidemic, however, particularly the organized efforts of the gay community, exerted a far more powerful influence than actions based on public health or medical science.

In 1983 and 1984, in New York State, Health Commissioner David Axelrod had to make an initial health policy decision about how to classify the new phenomenon of AIDS. Though this may look like a bureaucratic wrinkle, it in fact was very important. Presumably caused by an infectious agent and almost certainly transmissible by blood-borne and sexual means, AIDS would most naturally fit into one or more of the standard categories of communicable or sexually transmitted diseases. Diseases so listed under state public health law must be reported by physicians to the public health authorities. Further, in the loosely defined, outdated public health codes drafted early in the twentieth century, diseases in these categories carry connotations of mandatory testing and examination of "suspected" cases. They also required treatment and tracing of contacts (at government expense), and posed the potential for quarantine of infected individuals.

Because of concern by advocates (including most public health officers) that these provisions were inappropriate with AIDS, Axelrod did not wish to put AIDS in one of the traditional communicable disease categories. However, it was clearly necessary that cases of AIDS be reported to public health authorities so that the scope and evolution of the epidemic could be better understood.

Acting through the state Public Health Council, Axelrod adopted an ingenious course, labeling AIDS a one-of-a-kind reportable disease, in its own special category, with reporting of cases required to the state Health Department. In New York City, whose Health Department had its own separate statistics system, physicians reported cases of AIDS to the city Department of Health, which in turn transferred only statistical information (without any personal identifying information) to the state.

In all other areas of the state, the situation was the reverse: physicians reported directly to the state Health Department the names and relevant public health information of all persons diagnosed with AIDS, and the state Health Department informed the local (county) health officer only on a statistical basis. Thus the local health department found itself in the position of not being able to take any direct action such as targeted counseling or contact tracing even if it desired to do so, because it did not possess the names of those with a reportable disease. This anomalous system was constructed, of course, in the name of "preventing discrimination," but it crippled public health action in the upstate counties outside New York City.

It is unfortunate that the truly important signals sent by the early recognition of the dilemmas posed by AIDS classification were misread and not acted upon: the real issue was that outmoded public health law needed revision. Legislative action might have provided a clearer framework for more direct public health action, while retaining protection from abuses of individual rights. On the other hand, it is indeed possible that legislatures might well have overreacted, and rewritten or left standing public health statutes that would have been repressive in practice.

A sort of cosmetic compromise was adopted in New York and elsewhere, which served reasonably at first but became progressively inadequate as AIDS spread. The antibody test for asymptomatic infection became available in 1985. The dawn of specific therapy in 1987 made the early identification of infected individuals and the notification of their partners important. The special categorization of AIDS unfortunately also lent an aura of legitimacy to arguments that it was inappropriate to use traditional public health measures to warn individuals at risk and to slow the spread of the virus.

No issue surrounding the AIDS epidemic is more explosive than that of quarantining individuals who knowingly put others at risk of infection. The gay community sees in this the potential for concentration-camp roundups of homosexuals, and the indefinite imprisonment of individuals who have a lifelong, incurable infection.

Detention and quarantine have a long and firm place in the history of public health, as historical measures to protect the community from an infectious disease when transmission cannot be interrupted by other means, or in individuals who recklessly or even deliberately put others at risk of infection. In New York City, the saga of Typhoid Mary, who was a helpless carrier of the infection, and who would not remain away from food service work, has become a classic in public health because of her many years of incarceration on public health grounds. It is easy to see how, in the emotional context surrounding the AIDS epidemic, there should be deep fears among homosexuals that they would be singled out for mass repression. These fears are unfortunately fueled by the irresponsible statements of right-wing homophobes, and by the actions of countries such as Cuba, which has taken actual mass permanent detention measures against HIV-infected people.

And yet detention and quarantine are legitimate and important measures for the community to have in reserve, for self-protection when all else, and all lesser remedies, fail. A chief political executive or a health officer would be both foolish and derelict to renounce, a priori, any use of these measures.

The New York State and City Health Codes give Health Commissioners the power to make quarantine decisions in public health emergencies. The most usual cause of public health detention, which I invoked about a dozen times during my years as Health Commissioner, involves patients with active, infectious tuberculosis who refuse to take the medication that will, in addition to benefiting their own health, render them noninfectious to others. In a typical such case, the patient is kept, involuntarily if necessary, in the hospital until treatment results in noninfectiousness, or unless the patient gets a court injunction overturning the commissioner's order.

But tuberculosis and most other infectious diseases are quite different from AIDS. Treatment for tuberculosis is available as oral medication that can render the patient noninfectious to others in a matter of weeks; thus detention is time-limited. With HIV, of course, there is as yet no analogous treatment, and individuals are infectious to others for life. HIV depends upon conscious intimate behavior for transmission, while tuberculosis is more casually transmitted through the air. AIDS carries social stigmas far beyond other diseases—though this argument can be made too much of; we are only a generation or two removed from the time when tuberculosis, venereal disease, or cancer carried a stigma as powerful as that AIDS carries today.

In the usual course of events, individual or group quarantine for HIV infection is not justified. Its use would not only be ineffective, but would indeed drive those in need of diagnosis and services away from care. Since we have as yet no way to create noninfectiousness of HIV patients, detention would be inhumane and offensive because of its permanency.

And yet there are circumstances where considering detention or quarantine in the case of AIDS is warranted: those where an individual knowingly and repeatedly puts others at risk of this fatal infection, and where all lesser remedies such as education, psychotherapy or drug treatment, alternative employment or economic support, or threats of sanctions, have not led to cessation of risk behavior. In such a case (and one could cite compulsive or vindictive sexual behavior, or a deliberate attempt to pollute the blood supply—as happened in a case in California), I believe that society, acting through public health, has a right and a duty to protect itself, even at the price of depriving an individual of liberty. That seems to me inherent in the fundamental balance necessary for the protection of the public health.

Opponents of this position will say, at this point, that I am setting the stage for a "roundup of the prostitutes." Far from it; I would contest that we, as a society, have made virtually no efforts to provide AIDS education, alternative employment, or drug treatment to prostitutes (the majority of HIV-infected prostitutes are substance abusers).

I would argue that licensing, and strict medical supervision of prostitution is much preferable to the deadly consequences of public hypocrisy and neglect, especially in this time of sexually transmitted epidemic: a caveat emptor philosophy is not adequate preventive medicine.

The current reality of significant numbers of heavily infected, male transvestite prostitutes in New York City, their sexual identity at times unknown to their clients, poses a public health nightmare, and one which we have shrunk from addressing.

Would I be willing to invoke quarantine in an individual case of repeated and reckless endangerment of others, after lesser measures had been tried and had failed? Yes. Without hesitation. In attempting to strike that narrow balance between protection of the rights of the individual and the protection of the public health, I would put public health first.

But not in the traditional way of executive branch decision. I would apply for a court order, as the Health Department did when we closed five pornographic cinemas in New York City, where we had irrefutable evidence of commercially sanctioned, on premises, high-risk sexual activity. I would make my best case, and have the courts decide.

As I said in an op-ed on the subject of quarantine in the *New York Times:*

> If society wishes to restrict the power of public health officials, it could decide that such actions can only be taken with a prior court order. But there can be no doubt that the availability of these actions is necessary. While we must ensure that they are taken wisely and fairly, we must never renounce their availability.
>
> The issue, then, is not whether quarantine is a legitimate tool for protecting the public health. The issue is: under what circumstances should it be employed, and with what safeguards against its abuse. . . . Every New Yorker must realize that this issue cannot be decided rationally by street demonstrations by one self-interested group, or by sloganeering in political generalities. It is best decided by a combination of professional expertise, Mayoral leadership, and court oversight, acting on a case-by-case basis.

# Research and Knowledge

In the research arena, few would argue against continued investment in biomedical research. Research should remain focused on the nature and biological behavior of the HIVirus and on the development and testing of antiviral drugs. This approach, which has already yielded enormous payoff, will continue to have beneficial secondary effects on the crucial frontier of biomedicine where virology and immunology meet. The rewards here will go far beyond AIDS, and will open major lines of research to be pursued throughout the first half of the twenty-first century.

Basic and applied antiviral research should take priority over research aimed at opportunistic infections, though not by any means to their exclusion, because of the inevitable development of microbial resistance in infected people, and the inevitable substitution of one infection for another in the person with a damaged immune system.

The search for a vaccine must press on, and be given very high priority, but with a realistic understanding of its limitations for slowing the epidemic in the United States. An effective, safe, and low-cost vaccine offers the only feasible hope of reducing large-scale social catastrophe in Africa and other developing regions of the world.

Second in practical importance only to the development of a vaccine for primary prevention is the need to develop an effective drug, preferably administered orally, that would render an infected person noninfectious to others. Advances in this area, which has been relatively neglected in AIDS research to date, would be of the utmost value to public health efforts to slow the spread of HIV, especially when combined with other public health measures.

The greatest policy challenge to the rapid progress of AIDS research will be the growing arguments of other competitive research areas, including those such as heart disease and cancer, which have a very large and nationwide constituency. In what is almost certainly to be a time of fiscal restraint on the growth of research dollars in the economic climate of the early 1990s, protests that "AIDS is getting too much of the research pie" are likely to have considerable appeal to Congress and the American public.

These are difficult questions that no one enjoys facing, for every decision to do something implies a decision not to do something else. As available treatment for HIV illness gets more expensive and complex, and the numbers of surviving but severely affected people require vastly increased social services, the impact of AIDS on the health care sector will mount. It will be essential that we have some semblance of a longer range plan for what resources will be available and what services deployed.

It is particularly difficult to change policy rapidly in the health sector, where the training of personnel and the construction and equipping of facilities involves considerable time. Government regulation is so pervasive that even if a New York hospital wants to, say, build and equip a new wing, it cannot do so without passing an elaborate approval process by the state. The rationale is clear—protect the public from the costly overexpansion of hospitals—yet in practice the process is so onerous that it often serves as an impediment to good planning.

AIDS dramatized the cliché that an ounce of prevention is worth a pound of cure. By the end of the 1980s, federal investment in AIDS research exceeded the level of funds invested in heart disease research. Progress, thought extraordinarily rapid by any prior standard, seemed agonizingly and inexcusably slow to patients and their advocates.

Both the nation as a whole and individual states and communities need to plan ahead in a way that has so far not been accomplished. The various reports have produced thousands of recommendations, and have estimated billions of dollars in required costs, but there does not exist, to my knowledge, anywhere in the country, a local or state action plan that meshes policy, projected expenditures, and an approved multiyear timetable of funding and activities.

One of the most astonishing developments of the AIDS research story to date has been the effect AIDS advocates have had on the process of drug development, testing, and approval. Almost exclusively through their efforts, it has become apparent that many existing procedures are cumbersome and inadequate for meeting the needs of seriously ill people, especially those who have no therapeutic alternatives to experimental drugs. To date, this shaking of our confidence in the existing system has been a valuable development.

A careful evaluation should now be undertaken by an expert group, one that includes consumer representatives, about modifying laws and regulations governing drug development, approval, and availability in light of what AIDS has so far taught us. This should be a separate activity from the existing National Commission on AIDS, perhaps under the umbrella of the National Academy of Sciences' Institute of Medicine. The issue should be pursued in its broadest form, not just with respect to AIDS, with a view toward a reasoned overhaul of the existing federal machinery.

A scientifically sound system must be preserved; development, testing, and availability of new drugs cannot be done on the basis of who shouts loudest, nor exclusively according to short-range needs. The Food and Drug Administration, indeed the entire drug development and approval system, was set up in the first place to protect consumers from the kind of unscrupulous exploitation that remains a persistent danger—and it is important to remember that the flaws in a drug's safety and efficacy are often slow to reveal themselves.

The progress in research on the patterns of the epidemic, though seriously hampered by the unavailability of the up-to-date profiles of infection that would result from much more widespread antibody testing, has produced a good general understanding of the dynamics of the epidemic. We need to build further upon this, with more accurate profiles of current infection based on anonymous but also on confidential voluntary antibody testing, and to do this in an ongoing fashion and on a much greater scale.

This research needs to be tied much more closely than before to social science research, especially in the areas of sexual and drug abuse behavior. Such studies are notoriously difficult to do and to interpret, but we badly need improved understanding of the inter-relationships between sexual and drug behaviors and the movement of the virus between groups of people.

One area where more research is needed is on the effect of coun-seling and educational efforts on risk behavior. Little knowledge exists about what works, and why. Focused research in this area would be of great value to the future of AIDS prevention efforts.

Most of the sponsorship of the various areas of AIDS research will have to come from the federal government, though foundations have an important role in supporting studies that government finds too controversial.

Within each of the biomedical and epidemiologic research areas, coordination by the relevant federal agency (National Institutes of Health for the former, and the Centers for Disease Control for the latter) has been well managed. But very little coordination has oc-curred across the two areas, and so, for example, applied clinical research is not well tied to the critical epidemiologic studies that could best inform it. This poor coordination among diverse but mu-tually relevant research areas is compounded by the low quality of much of the federally funded research in drug abuse.

# Treatment

While all these conflicts over appropriate prevention activities were evolving, the ferment was, if anything, greater on the treat-ment side of the issues.

Possibilities for treatment of HIV infection developed with a slight lag behind the prevention controversies. In the first years of the epidemic, the most important fact about treatment was that there wasn't any; physicians and patients in North America were faced with a specter that had been avoided for a generation or more: a major outbreak of a progressive and fatal infectious disease against which there was absolutely nothing but general supportive care. Nothing similar had been experienced since the recurrent epidemics of the nineteenth century and the influenza pandemic at the end of the First World War. Perhaps only older physicians, who had worked during the polio outbreaks of the 1940s and 1950s, had an adequate standard of reference for the helpless position that medicine found itself in.

The sophisticated diagnostic capability of contemporary biomedicine was quick to understand the nature of the opportunistic infections, but the large majority of them were caused by agents against which no standard therapy existed. Against the AIDS virus itself, we had absolutely no weapons. AIDS represented the frontier where immunology intersects with virology; this was a therapeutic frontier that had not been crossed, and only crudely mapped.

In the first several years of the epidemic, a typical pattern of diagnosis was one in which a young man was rushed to the hospital critically ill with respiratory distress, was diagnosed as having pneumonia, spent a horrific period of days or weeks in the intensive care unit, and died without ever leaving the hospital.

This pattern gradually became less common over the next few years as patients appeared for care in earlier stages of HIV illness, as diagnostic accuracy increased, as general supportive care for the problems of AIDS became more sophisticated, and therapy against the opportunistic infections and the HIVirus itself was devised. By 1987, in New York City, gay men were surviving for a median period of almost two years after diagnosis. Drug addicts and women were surviving for significantly shorter periods, most likely because of later diagnosis of illness and less access to complex and costly supportive care.

Reams of argument and counterargument have been written concerning the quality and adequacy of the effort by research scientists, government, and the pharmaceutical industry to develop more effective therapy against AIDS. One extreme position, held by some AIDS activists and journalists, is that there was negligence, incompetence, and venality that hobbled research and accessibility of treatment to the extent of criminality.

My own view, expressed throughout this book, is that the reality was, and is, quite different: the speed and effective application of resources with which therapy was developed was unprecedented given the complexity of the problem. Perhaps the medical miracles of the twentieth century had led us to discount the awesome power of dragons, and to misunderstand the feebleness of our defenses against them.

AIDS is teaching important lessons that should be explored and acted on, that will in the end leave the biomedical system more effective and more equable than before. The effort to develop AIDS therapy, with all its large and small flaws, has been magnificent.

As the toll of illness, and the projections of much higher burdens to come, mounted in New York, it became apparent that health care resources would be strained and perhaps overwhelmed. Health Department projections of 20,000 cumulative AIDS cases by 1988, 30,000 by 1990, and 60,000 by 1993, projections that continue to prove accurate, left no doubt of the strains to come upon the system. Beyond the AIDS case numbers lay a daunting series of care needs: for people with HIV illness not meeting the AIDS criteria, for a range of medical, dental, mental health, social service, and human support needs that in scale surpassed any prior challenge.

In New York City, the stresses were compounded by the burdens of poverty. In a population of almost eight million, 40 percent of the children lived below the poverty line. The city had only recently emerged from the fiscal crisis of the late 1970s, and was soon to enter the very severe financial crisis of the early 1990s. It was beset by mammoth problems on all sides: homelessness (estimated at more than 45,000 persons in the late 1980s), a vicious and persistent drug abuse epidemic (with 200,000 heroin addicts whose numbers were soon to be swollen, perhaps doubled, by the crack explosion), a severe shortage of low- and middle-income housing, crumbling public sector systems of education and hospital care, an overburdened court system, a mushrooming prison population, loss of public confidence in the ability of the police to keep the citizenry safe from violent criminals, and an increasingly ugly climate of racial and ethnic antagonism. This in the face of federal policy of the 1980s which abandoned the cities to their fates.

In the sea of New York's troubles, AIDS was just one more rock dropped into the waves. The city administration was slow to recognize the dimensions of the AIDS crisis, or to directly involve itself in aggressive education of the public. As late as mid-1985, the Mayor's closest health advisor was repeatedly quoted as stating, "There is no AIDS crisis. Everything is under control." Gay advocacy groups began early and persistently to criticize the city's slow response. But the real dilemmas lay not in prevention, but in the availability of treatment.

When I began to make my case, in mid-1986, to the Mayor and to the public, for an increased recognition of the seriousness of the epidemic and for hugely increased resources to combat it, I found Ed Koch to be steadily supportive. Here, of course, the resources required were only a small fraction of the dollar costs of health treatment and social services. Despite the city's budget-cutting, our Health Department budget for AIDS prevention doubled each year between 1987 and 1990.

My assets in fighting for increased resources were the increasing public concern, the growing power of AIDS advocates who were often my allies and yet increasingly my adversaries, the basic inclination of the Mayor to accept the technical advice of his Health Commissioner, and all the tenacity and energy I could muster in the budget struggles. My adversaries were the green-eyeshades in the Office of Management and Budget (who, as staff gnomes, are the same the world over, one-eyed and coldly arrogant), and the impossibly difficult competing demands for resources needed for urgent problems in multiple sectors. The price that we had to pay for budget increases for AIDS and related areas (such as tuberculosis and sexually transmitted diseases) was to accept cuts in other public health programs. The strength and scope of our AIDS public health programs grew rapidly. We could have done more, of course. We always could have done more, all of us, and that will continue to be the case until we finally begin to get ahead of the virus. That day is still far away.

What seemed to me most important to do as Health Commissioner was to keep driving the process, to never let AIDS out of the public consciousness or the government machinery, to hammer and claw away for every additional increment of money and public awareness. The reality was that public health advances in AIDS are measured by successive inches, and that no bright angel is going to arrive with the magic arrow. AIDS is trench warfare.

Even before, but especially after, the beginning of specific therapy with AZT in 1987, the strains on the New York hospitals were extraordinary. The number of beds taken up by HIV-ill patients on a daily basis was 1,100 in late 1986, then 1,400 six months later, and some 1,900 by late 1989. During the same period, the drug epidemic placed an even greater strain on the capacity of the hospitals.

In the early 1980s, New York City appeared, along with most of the rest of the country, to have excess hospital bed capacity that was wasteful in a rapidly inflating health sector. Using the broad regulatory powers available to him, State Health Commissioner David Axelrod set about trimming the apparent fat. Hospitals in the city were closed, wards were taken out of service, and the entire system was reduced. The problem is that the health sector is inelastic and slow to respond to changes of need and demand. This is especially true of hospitals, which take a long time to build or renovate, equip, and staff.

By the mid-1980s the twin epidemics of drugs and AIDS had swamped the city's shrunken hospital base, particularly the public hospitals, which were fast in danger of becoming "AIDS and drugs hospitals." Daily bed occupancy rates, a comfortable or even slack 75–85 percent in other cities, were in the high 90s or even over 100 percent in New York City hospitals. In a drastic summer and fall of 1988, the city was stunned by the routine occurrence of patients waiting for four or five days on stretchers in emergency rooms before a hospital bed became available; there were predictions of imminent chaos in the system.

The policies of 1980 were clearly overtaken by the realities of the later years of the decade. Health Commissioner Axelrod resisted relaxing the constraints. In his often expressed view, "there was still plenty of fat in the system," and no reason to release the pressure. He did eventually approve a small increment of additional beds for

AIDS, but these were very slow in coming into service because of fiscal constraints on the hospitals and the long processes of regulatory approval. More usefully, Axelrod created enhanced state reimbursement rates to hospitals for AIDS care, thus pumping money and incentive into the system.

But he refused to agree to increased hospital beds. This, plus the rapidly escalating fiscal crises by 1990 and beyond, dealt a final blow to any possibility that the city would be able to develop the hospital resources to cope adequately with the AIDS burden.

As the 1980s progressed, three factors were making more complex the range and quantity of needs. The first was, of course, the growth in the size of the epidemic. But beyond this was our expanding understanding of the full range of HIV illness—far beyond the standard diagnosis of AIDS.

In 1988 and 1989, the important benefits of early diagnosis and treatment became evident. The number of persons in need of access to medically effective services in New York City suddenly skyrocketed from the 6,000 or so living people diagnosed with full-blown AIDS. The 25,000 people living with lesser forms of HIV illness could now be helped with early treatment, to prevent opportunistic infections and to delay the progression of their underlying disease. Further, some unknown but very large proportion (perhaps half) of the 200,000 or so HIV-infected individuals, most of whom were asymptomatic, and most of whom did not even know they were infected, also became eligible by newer medical criteria for early intervention.

Second, the increasing proportion among the HIV-ill of people who were drug users, poor, and black or Hispanic, placed an ever-increasing service burden onto the publicly financed sector, with dire consequences for both the fiscal health and quality of care available.

And third, AIDS was deeply embedded in the major social problems of the city: the homeless mentally ill, the drug epidemic, the faltering public education system. Health and social service needs related to AIDS were necessary across a much, much broader front than had earlier been contemplated.

In 1988, New York City spent $1 billion on the AIDS epidemic.

Between 1989 and 1993, the direct costs of services for the epidemic are projected to run to a cumulative $7 billion.

Even if this amount of money were to be made available, and even if the other demands of a city in crisis were stabilized, there would be great uncertainty that the necessary range of service and support systems could be put in place promptly.

We will not see treatment services adequate to the need during the coming height of the epidemic in New York City. There will be a period, during the mid- and late-1990s, when city services, particularly health and hospital services, may collapse. The inevitable result of this pressure will be a marked drop in the accessibility and quality of *all* health and social services, not just those related directly to AIDS, nor exclusively those provided in the public sector. The great task will be to keep the health system running with some assurance that critical needs will be met.

Could the city have done more, earlier, to expand services and access to care? Yes, certainly, but only at the margin. An earlier development of expanded outpatient primary care for those with HIV illness would have positioned us better now that specific therapy is becoming available. But a significant investment in that area would have meant reductions for other needs in the hard-pressed public hospitals and clinics—tradeoffs whose legitimacy is far from clear. Can the city expand and improve the quality of AIDS care rapidly? Again, I am doubtful that more than marginal improvement will be possible, especially given the financial climate that all levels of government face in the early 1990s.

This convergence between prevention and treatment dilemmas leads to an inescapable conclusion: every future case of AIDS that can be prevented will reduce the burdens that have to be borne; every lost opportunity to prevent a case of AIDS extends and increases the length and cost of the road yet to be traveled. The three most important challenges to meet in facing the epidemic are: prevention, prevention, and prevention.

# What We Need to Do Now

*The federal government must lead the war against AIDS.* If the federal government can be said to have done a credible job of funding AIDS research, and a mediocre one of mobilizing public awareness and education, it did an inadequate job in assisting the states with the financing of needed health and social services for AIDS. The 1990 passage of the Kennedy-Waxman ("Ryan White") bill may be the first indication of a change. The bill provides for federal assistance for the direct provision of services by states and the most affected cities. However, as of 1992, the appropriation under the bill was far below the authorized level. Rather than the current piecemeal approach, it would be far better to have a national strategy on AIDS, approved by Congress, covering the wide range of issues that will have to be faced—manpower, facilities, insurance, costs of services, types and organization of services, as well as the many prevention and education issues.

If only to prevent vital public sector services in some areas from going under, the federal government will have to contribute substantially to paying for AIDS services. But it should use this opportunity to insist on improved effectiveness and cost efficiency. For example, experience in New York and San Francisco shows that the emphases in AIDS treatment should be: long-term care, home health services, primary care, and closer coordination of medical, nursing, and social services than usually exist. Federal dollars can move care in these directions.

Similarly, as a condition for federal funding, states should require all physicians to provide evidence of continuing education in the basics of HIV diagnosis and management. Many states already have requirements for continuing education as prerequisites for licensing, as do most medical specialty associations. These should include AIDS education so that the current generation of physicians is up to speed in what is a virtually new and undeniably critical area of medicine.

As the pressures of the epidemic mount, even larger burdens will fall on hospitals that serve the inner-city poor. The most successful method of treating large numbers of adult HIV-ill patients in hospitals has been the AIDS-designated service ward, where specialized knowledge and intensely dedicated staff can be concentrated. Most observers have felt that separate "AIDS-designated hospitals" are not a good idea, that they would exacerbate discrimination, tend to gravitate toward lower funding, and have difficulty in recruiting and retaining staff. At the extreme of this argument lies the specter of the Dickensian workhouse. I agree with the dangers pointed to by those opposed to special-purpose hospitals for AIDS, but I am not confident that we will be able to avoid their creation—in New York and perhaps in one or two other hardest hit cities.

*Cities must plan concretely for treatment.* If we continue to fail to plan and enforce an equitable distribution of HIV-ill patients among all hospitals in the community, if we fail to provide the increase in available hospital beds that will be needed to cope with the epidemic (estimated at between 4,000 and 5,000 beds in New York City by the mid-1990s, or almost 20 percent of the city's existing hospital beds), then it is highly probable that we will be forced to create new and separate facilities. Rather than being forced, unprepared, to do this at the eleventh hour, we would be far better advised to plan ahead for the hospital care of large numbers of chronically ill patients who require sophisticated levels of medical technology, at very high cost.

In New York, this means facing the need to develop one or two AIDS-dedicated facilities—either separate hospitals or, much more preferable, large wings of existing general hospitals—to act as a buffer to the enormous load the general hospitals will have to face. The aim should be to set a standard of excellence in the specialized care of HIV illness. These HIV-designated facilities should be closely connected with general hospitals, and with extended care/nursing home resources.

It is highly unlikely that we will discover easy solutions to providing adequate HIV health care services. But applying the same remedies to AIDS that have thus far applied to the larger health system —piecemeal tinkering, political indecisiveness, sustained unfairness, and runaway costs—will produce a recipe for disaster.

*Education about risk was the earliest weapon in the epidemic, and must continue.* The 1990s will require that several critical messages reach several critical groups. First, it would be a great mistake to think that efforts at risk reduction among gay men can slacken; if anything, they must accelerate. The hardest to reach—closeted gays and bisexuals, those with the strongest sense of denial, and young men who think that AIDS was a passing threat of the 1980s, are still out there in large numbers. The maintenance of safer-sex behavior is eroding. Gay community groups, in particular, need to further evolve the effective educational campaigns that they mounted early in the epidemic into messages for the long haul.

Second, IV drug users remain beyond our effective reach. But to the concentration on the drug injector must be added a more difficult concentration on people who abuse drugs by other means, and on the sexual behavior of both groups. There is no current reason for optimism about effecting changes in sexual behavior of drug addicts, though we must keep trying. We must also place the maximum stress on the prevention of drug abuse itself, through a wide range of educational, treatment, and law enforcement measures. Despite its weaknesses, the current system of drug treatment needs major expansion linked to systems of primary health care and HIV counseling and testing.

*Needle exchange programs should be strongly supported, especially in cities with high concentrations of poverty and large numbers of shooting galleries.* Needle exchange offers the best hope of a bridge to drug treatment, bringing addicts into contact with rehabilitative services, helping them make the transition into drug treatment, and reducing HIV transmission risks for those who cannot get access to, or will not get, treatment. To deny this combined therapeutic and public health approach to those who need it on the basis of shopworn shibboleths about "promoting drug use" is both unconscionable and foolish.

The most critical area of AIDS education in the 1990s involves minority communities. These efforts are fraught with hazard in that they are likely to be labeled (indeed, already have been in many instances) discriminatory or racist in implication. But the increasing concentration of the epidemic among poor blacks and Hispanics is a public health crisis, and the need is urgent to provide protection as effectively and rapidly as possible.

*The leadership of minority communities—political, religious, and popular figures—must take a frank position on AIDS education and prevention.* Substantial public funding should go to community-based groups that can be effective at education and prevention. Gay advocacy groups have provided a clear example of how well this approach can work, and minority communities would do well to emulate it.

School systems have done a tepid job of AIDS education with rhetoric outpacing actual classroom teaching by a wide margin. One way to change that is for concerned parents' groups to press for AIDS education. In many school districts, joint AIDS education of children and their parents could be very useful, not only for increasing knowledge, but for reducing anxiety and discrimination.

Adolescents will represent a slowly increasing but particularly dangerous segment of the HIV-infected population. Infection of young adolescents who are experimenting with drugs or sex will provide a source of new infections, especially in urban settings, unconnected with known traditional risk behavior. This involves those who are approaching their most intense period of sexual activity, with the possibility of many partners over a decade or more. Active programs of AIDS and drug abuse education beginning in the primary schools represent the best method of protecting our children.

We should understand, however, that the high-risk street kids, runaway and "throwaway" youth, are unlikely to be effectively reached by school-based efforts. For these adolescents, street-based services provided by organizations that gain their trust are the only feasible approach to prevention, early diagnosis, and treatment. AIDS activities for street kids should be combined with other health and social services and shelter, which have greater apparent and immediate value to youth in daily search of survival.

AIDS education messages also need to evolve significantly in the 1990s. To date, the basic message has been some version of "Protect yourself." This will remain an indispensable theme, but increasingly we need to add a second theme: "Consider AIDS antibody testing, know your partners, and seek treatment early if you are infected."

*The media must cover the epidemic accurately and courageously.* Journalists are often criticized, especially by gay advocacy groups, for ignoring or downplaying AIDS in the early years of the epidemic. I believe this criticism has been overdrawn. Certainly, there was a reluctance to cover what was perceived to be a story affecting homosexuals and drug users. There was, unfortunately, significant homophobia and fear of infection among many news organizations. For example, I was told while recording broadcasts at New York City radio stations even in the late 1980s that technicians (and some guests) refused to use microphones and chairs in recording studios after a person with AIDS, until the room had been "disinfected." As late as 1988, one of the New York TV network affiliate stations had only a single camera crew that would go out to cover AIDS stories, because of the technicians' fear of casual contagion! Yet this distancing was not restricted to the media, but generalized throughout the population. I think journalists did a better job than most (although editors of the *New York Times* could not bring themselves to print the words "gay man" until 1986 or to list AIDS as a cause of death in an obituary until 1987).

In addition, the AIDS story was scientifically complex. AIDS is certainly a process rather than an event, and the media do not do as well with process stories, especially within the constraints of the thirty-second sound bite. Further, there was much uncertainty over just what many of the "facts" actually were, especially in the first years of the epidemic.

After the sensationalism over the illness and death of Rock Hudson in 1985, the media provided intense and continuing coverage of AIDS. In New York City, as familiarity with the issues evolved, both print and electronic media began to offer generally accurate and responsible coverage. This was especially so in those cases where a full-time reporter was assigned to the beat, or where regular feature writers began to do in-depth explorations of the epidemic. Similarly, there was no lack of editorial commentary on the public policy issues that surfaced as the epidemic evolved.

The criticism that I do believe valid, especially with regard to the tabloid newspapers and television, is that they played too often to the sensational, and were unwilling or unable to distinguish and articulate the shades of uncertainty that formed the reality of AIDS. There were many mornings when I rather expected to see the front page of the New York *Post* proclaiming, "Martians Land with AIDS." Perhaps the lack of a photograph deterred them.

*We must face the difficult task of removing the fear that has grown up around the antibody test, and begin to employ it to its full benefit:* for all persons at potential risk, for couples considering childbearing, for pregnant women, for patients in hospitals or with unclear diagnosis.

Antibody testing should remain voluntary and the results confidential, but strong efforts must be made for both public and professional acceptance of the routine use of the antibody test. Existing systems of counseling in connection with the test have been designed emphasizing the dangers to the individual of possible breaches of confidentiality. These are undeniable, but they have been stressed to the detriment of the advantages of early diagnosis of infection. Procedures for counseling and written informed consent have been overly cumbersome, and have inhibited the widespread use of the test. All of this now needs to be streamlined, demystified, and combined with federal and state legislation that mandates strong protection of confidentiality of HIV-related information, yet also encourages testing and allows information to be used medically to protect against further infection or to provide appropriate care for those already infected.

Another group who should be given added attention in AIDS education is one that is usually not considered: health workers. Doctors, nurses, and other health professionals need to be counseled about their own risks and the risks to others. The number of HIV-infected health care personnel, though very small in an absolute sense, will continue to rise; health workers will be at increasing risk as HIV infection becomes less obviously tied to traditional risk behaviors. Cases of AIDS in health professionals will continue to draw attention and anxiety far out of proportion to their number, and the extremely rare cases of transmission of infection from professional to patient, which will undoubtedly occur, may shake public confidence to a surprising degree.

Transmission of HIV infection from patients to health care workers and from health care workers to patients are two edges of the same sharp sword. Both are very unlikely, though both can and have occurred. Both cause profound anxiety and dread in any group that fears it might be infected (such as trauma surgeons in inner-city hospitals, or patients who think their dentist is gay). Both give rise to situations where discrimination has serious consequences, such as the loss of a doctor's practice or the refusal to treat patients thought to be at risk or infected.

In neither case is it feasible to mandate HIV testing of all patients or all health workers. Such policies would overload the laboratory systems for small numbers of positive results. But it would be reasonable to urge antibody testing for all patients who might be thought at risk (such as all pregnant women in high-prevalence areas, or all patients with a sexual history that is assessed as being at risk). It is not unreasonable to argue for "routine" antibody testing, as long as the patient knows what is being done, and has the right to refuse the test.

"Universal precautions" that reduce the risk of blood-to-blood contact in the operating room should remain standard procedure for *all* patients, and patients who refuse testing should be treated with special care (though not with neglect). Vigorous and aggressive routine urging by physicians to their patients who present any risk factors (including geographic residence) to be tested is a far preferable course to blanket mandatory testing.

As for physicians and other health workers who perform invasive procedures, it would be impractical in the extreme to mandate universal and frequent testing. The problem of patient safety (and remember, we are talking here of very, very low risk, with extremely low probability of infection of patients by physicians) can best be addressed by considering the following:

First, there can be no question but that the health professional who believes that he is infected or at risk of infection has an obligation to know his actual status and to communicate the fact of his infection to patients. No matter how small the risk of transmission, it is the patient who has the right of informed consent, not the physician. Some will argue that this is only so if the physician (or other health worker) performs "invasive procedures." I would argue that this is too limited, both because of uncertainty over what constitutes an invasive procedure, and because of the patient's right to set his own comfort level. Will this bring real (and sometimes unjustified) hardship upon some physicians? Yes. Is there a better way to draw the line? I don't think so.

Hospital staff committees and professional societies should be vigorous in enforcing this policy. They, and the rest of society, must also find ways to compensate and otherwise employ the health professionals who lose their practice.

Second, we need to reach some reasonable understanding of what actually constitutes invasive procedures, and what the transmission risks associated with them are. This is very difficult, especially because the risks of actual transmission here are so small. The best approach would be to have a set of general national guidelines, perhaps formulated by the Centers for Disease Control, which should be interpreted in detail at the local level by a committee that includes health professionals and lay persons from a variety of fields, much as the earlier groups that decided on patients' suitability for kidney dialysis or transplantation in the early days of those procedures.

There is no absolute way to totally protect against the greatest fears here: that patients and doctors will hide the fact of their infections from each other, and that doctors will flee from service in areas of high prevalence of AIDS. But these are the same fears (and to some extent realities) that have been present in all the great plagues; they cannot be dealt with by blinding ourselves to them, and they can only be dealt with by hedging the bets strongly in favor of honesty.

Two groups of clinicians had early and continuing contact with AIDS. One group consisted of those physicians in high-prevalence areas who had private practices that included large numbers of gay men. These doctors—some of whom were themselves homosexual, and not a few of whom became AIDS patients—bore the early, most bewildering, and most frustrating medical burden, as increasing numbers of their patients sickened and died. Most of these physicians and a small number of dentists continued doing their heroic work through the first decade of the epidemic. A few burned out on the constant and rising tide of the deaths of young patients, a context of helplessness unfamiliar to most North American physicians. We should have great respect for those who did this exhausting and emotionally draining work, and should honor the memory of those who pressed on while themselves falling ill and dying of AIDS.

The second group of clinicians bearing the brunt of the epidemic were those caring for hospitalized indigent AIDS patients, increasingly minority drug users. There were without doubt many instances of discrimination against AIDS (or suspected AIDS) patients even in the settings where they were most frequently met with, especially in the earliest days when there was most doubt about risk from casual contact. But future observers will judge the record of those medical institutions that bore the brunt of the burden to have been truly outstanding. While there is not much reason to expect that the personnel of these institutions would have had very different attitudes and stereotypes about homosexuals or drug users than the rest of their colleagues and society in general, the important lesson is that those who were most directly exposed to the tangible clinical pressures of the epidemic were least likely to desert their responsibilities. Calls for withholding medical care or irrational measures for "protection" of hospital personnel were much more likely to come from rural medical societies or surgeons at private midwestern hospitals than from house staff or attending physicians at New York's Bellevue or Harlem Hospital or San Francisco General.

For all health personnel, but especially for doctors and nurses, the AIDS epidemic created a major shift in the sense of personal vulnerability. Before AIDS, decades had passed since physicians worried seriously about contracting an untreatable case of tuberculosis or blood poisoning while caring for patients. Despite the possibilities of infection with the hepatitis virus, the vast majority of physicians and nurses had felt themselves to be free of personal risk in the practice of their profession.

AIDS changed all that. Especially as risks of occupational exposure became more apparent, medical personnel have had to come to grips with their own mortality. Yet despite some instances of self-interested behavior at the expense of patients, the record of physicians, nurses, and allied health professionals has been one of which we can be extraordinarily proud.

We are standing at a moment in the AIDS epidemic when we have what may be our last opportunity to stem a further major wave of ongoing infection: of minority heterosexuals in the urban areas, and of gay men and drug users in the smaller cities and suburban and rural areas where infection is currently of less intensity.

Education and advocacy for risk reduction remain important tools in this effort but, alone, they will never accomplish the objective: to make a difference at last in the speed and extent of the virus's spread. This can only be achieved by combining educational and early intervention efforts with specific measures guiding those resources to the people who need them most: those who are already infected, and to their sex and drug partners.

Those specific measures are the time-proven public health tools of mandatory confidential reporting of infection, and the tracing of contacts of those who have been reported as infected. These measures have been portrayed, largely by gay activists, as repressive invasions of civil liberties, one step removed from a wholesale police roundup of infected persons. In reality, they are public health tools that are routinely used, every day, with immense benefits in a wide variety of circumstances. These include such disparate areas as containment of measles outbreaks, combating the spread of meningitis in daycare centers, and in highly successful public health campaigns of the past against tuberculosis and syphilis. Like all public policy tools, they are vulnerable to possible abuse, but the instances of their misuse by public health officials in this country are minimal.

The availability of increasingly effective early treatment of HIV infection and its opportunistic infections add urgency to the need to find and warn those at special risk as well as those already infected.

The availability of drugs to reduce the infectiousness of an HIV-infected person will affect the epidemic only if infected individuals can be identified.

Contact tracing as employed in public health is a confidential voluntary process conducted by trained public health investigators, who interview persons infected with disease $x$ (classically, patients treated for a sexually transmitted disease), ascertaining from them the names of other persons who either might have infected the initial case or might have been infected by the initial case. The patient is assured that the contacts will not be told the identity of the person identifying them. Even with a mutually monogamous couple, the trained VD investigator will never name the partner who identified the other.

The chain of infection is traced ever wider. All traced contacts (not all contacts are found) are urged to undertake testing or diagnosis for disease $x$. Contacts who turn out to be infected receive the individual and public health benefits of early treatment, and in turn lead to further contacts. Contacts who prove to be negative for infection nonetheless present an opportunity for preventive education —by definition, they are high-risk persons.

The benefits of such a system, vigorously pursued, for slowing HIV transmission in areas of low prevalence, where there are a relatively small number of contacts to trace and infected individuals to identify, are obvious.

In the large urban areas of high intensity of HIV infection, and with high rates of drug use, prostitution, and multiple partners, opponents have argued that contact tracing would not be cost effective. In truth, quite the opposite is the case. Of course one would not attempt to trace every single sexual partner or needle-sharing companion over the course of the past ten years; one would, on the contrary, selectively try to locate the contacts of highest risk of the patients at highest risk.

For example, the New York City Medical Examiner looked at a large sample of dead persons who were tested postmortem and found to be HIV-positive, but who had no notation in their medical records of having been diagnosed as infected. Over 35 percent of those persons had a readily identifiable spouse or steady sexual partner. How can one justify, on clinical, public health, or humanitarian grounds, *not* notifying that surviving partner, who might be the source of the infection in the deceased, or the recipient of infection? Arguments against this procedure border on the absurd; one has to start with the premise that increased medical knowledge is more dangerous than helpful to the individual, and that the rights of the uninfected count for nothing against the rights of the infected.

Vigorous contact tracing, under conditions of strict public health confidentiality, is the most important step we can now take to reduce the further progress of the HIVirus, and to protect those who, unsuspecting, are at greatest risk of infection or in greatest need of early medical management.

In order to be effective on a population-based scale, contact tracing needs to be combined with mandatory reporting by physicians to the public health authority, under conditions of strict confidentiality, of those persons who are infected with the virus. The public health authority can then decide, utilizing the physician's advice, that either (1) the index case has notified his/her own partners; (2) the physician has undertaken such notification; or (3) the health department should undertake an interview and contact investigation.

Mandatory reporting also would have the benefit of giving a far more accurate and up-to-date pattern of the epidemic, locality by locality. There is neither need nor reason to have a national system of named reporting; public health action is taken at the state and local level, and statistical reporting with anonymity of individuals is all that is necessary for federal epidemiologic purposes.

Mandatory reporting, especially combined with a massive expansion of voluntary confidential antibody testing, is the strategic underpinning to contact tracing. Those who see in it a specter of government repression ignore its widespread use in public health for everything from chicken pox to tuberculosis to lead poisoning— thirty-four diseases and conditions are currently reportable by law in New York City, with major benefits to the protection of the individual as well as to the wider community.

The record of public health in keeping such material confidential is outstanding in the United States. In New York City, as in most of the rest of the country, a clinical diagnosis of AIDS was mandatory for physicians to report to the Health Department from the earliest days of the epidemic. Without this information we would have been flying completely blind in understanding and combating the epidemic. The New York City Department of Health kept that information under the strictest lock and key; only those epidemiologists actually working with the information had access to it. Epidemiologic information passed on to state and federal health agencies contained no identifying names.

This list of names reached 30,000 by the winter of 1990. There was never a single leak or breach of confidentiality from that system, even when we were directly threatened by court action in individual cases, nor even in the early and more sensationalist days of the epidemic. (I had made special technical arrangements to hide, from the city's own lawyers, epidemiologic data pertaining to an HIV-infected physician who was suing the City of New York. I, and most other Health Commissioners, I am sure, would have chosen to go to jail on contempt of court charges rather than release this confidential Department of Health information that was being sought by the Corporation Counsel. Fortunately, my stonewalling prevailed, and the city's lawyers backed off from their demands.) In the 1990s, the need to know, in confidential public health terms, the names of the HIV-infected is analogous to the 1980s need to know the names of those diagnosed with AIDS. The record of public health agencies on the latter should provide reassurance for the former.

The hour is late, and the dragon has been long within the gates. But we all—public health professionals, individuals and groups most at risk, and the larger society and its leadership—have only ourselves to blame if we do not take the actions, and especially the range of vigorous preventive measures, that will give us the best bulwark possible against the continued growth of this tragedy. There is much that we can still salvage, both for the welfare of individuals (at risk, or already infected) and for the welfare of the entire community.

I believe that future generations will view with a certain measure of contempt those who understood this equation, yet failed to act.

# 3

## *The Politics of AIDS: The Gay Community*

There is no such thing as safe sex.

—John Cardinal O'Connor, Archdiocese of New York

I would always want to remember gay people loving each other and having a wonderful time, because they didn't have fear of AIDS. Fire Island expressed itself as being the forerunner of everything, be it design, be it style, be it fashion, be it excessive sex. We were young. We were all beautiful.

—HIV-positive gay man

THE HIVIRUS, SMART VIRUS THAT IT IS, HAS ADOPTED AN EVOLUTIONARY strategy that is both effective and efficient.

Microorganisms that injure or kill the host they infect have two possible pathways to success—success being defined as the increase and survival of their species.

One pathway has been chosen by organisms that are highly infectious and easily transmissible from one individual host to another. These organisms may cause severe illness, even rapid death, but they rely on mass infectiousness and casual and rapid communicability for evolutionary survival. The viruses that cause measles, influenza, and smallpox are examples of such evolutionary strategies, as are those which, at a lower level of life-threatening illness, are responsible for chicken pox and the common cold (see chart on page 88). The measles virus is so infectious that if a nonimmune person gets on a bus carrying a person who is infected and coughing, the nonimmune person's chances of becoming infected (and passing the virus onto others) are almost 100 percent. In evolutionary terms, measles was extremely successful—at least until the development of a protective vaccine. Today's middle-aged adults can remember how every schoolchild, without exception, contracted measles.

In Africa, and other poor regions of the world, measles is a disease of preschool, rather than school-age, children, and in pre-vaccine settings massive epidemics swept through localities every two or three years, as a "new crop" of susceptible children appeared. Mortality is as high as 10 percent in some of these epidemics, especially where early childhood malnutrition is rife.

The other major route to evolutionary success, for a disease-causing microorganism, is more complicated, involving a lower degree of infectiousness, but an infection that persists in the living host for a long time. Malaria and many other parasitic infections fall into this category. Many such parasites live a complicated life cycle, moving through other life forms as intermediate hosts, hosts which usually do not die but also cannot rid themselves of the invader until that invader moves on to the next host species in its natural cycle.

### CHARACTERISTICS OF SOME INFECTIOUS DISEASES

|  | Ease of Transmission | Chronicity of Infection, Length of Infectious Period |
|---|---|---|
| Measles: | very high | low, short |
| Common Cold: | very high | low, short |
| Malaria: | relatively low | relatively high |
| Tuberculosis: | intermediate to high | high, long |
| HIV: | low | very high |

HIVirus is one example of this slow but persistent approach. It is not a terribly explosive infection—or it would rapidly kill off its host population, with no one left to infect, and no insurance for survival of the virus. HIV has a difficult time getting from one person to another but once it makes it, its new host survives for a long time. What is more, the infected person remains infectious to other people for ten years or more, in contrast to the few days during which a person with measles is infectious to others. Tuberculosis, as an another example, produces an infection that can remain communicable to others over a long period which sometimes extends over several decades. It is not uncommon for a TB-infected individual to "break down" and become infectious to others many years after the initial infection, long after "cure" was thought to have taken place.

The evolutionary niche carved out for itself by HIV is an example of superb adaptation, one in which slow but sure transmission, lifelong infection, and prolonged survival of the infectious host are advantageous to the virus. Thus, the future major patterns of AIDS transmission are virtually certain to remain within its traditional boundaries.

Knowing the precise characteristics of any invading virus or bacteria is crucial to developing effective strategies of prevention and medical treatment. What became fundamental in the case of the AIDS epidemic was that these biological understandings of the nature of the virus took second place—a distant second place—to the politics of the epidemic.

The politics of AIDS defined AIDS well before any detailed medical definition took hold. AIDS is the first major public health issue in this century for which political values rather than health requirements set the agenda. The political definition of the epidemic— defined first by gay men and later modified by a stream of civil libertarians and political spokesmen—drove and determined the medical and public health response until well after the epidemic was in full flower.

All significant public health issues have powerful social and political dimensions—these are part of the essence of public health—but in no other issue in modern times have these factors so directly defined the problem and society's response to it.

In part this was due to the context of the times, which were highly influenced by the civil rights, consumer, and women's movements of the 1960s and 1970s. In particular, the homosexual community asserted its primacy both in defining the epidemic and establishing the yardsticks by which responses to the epidemic were judged—yardsticks of gay identity, autonomy, and expressions of sexuality.

Further, the nature of the medical and epidemiologic puzzles of AIDS were partly responsible for the passivity of public health and medicine, which were following, rather than leading, political concepts. Fairly soon after the epidemic was recognized in 1982, researchers knew (or had strong and ultimately correct hypotheses about) the viral cause; the means of transmission and associated risk factors; and, to some extent, the cycle of infection and illness concerned with the human immunodeficiency virus. But for several years neither a specific treatment nor even any specific means of prevention existed.

From another perspective, AIDS is the first truly modern epidemic, and presages important future trends. Its definition in political and social terms (so politically successful that taboo behaviors were to a significant extent redefined as acceptable), the astonishing speed with which basic science and applied medicine and public health began to solve its riddles, the powerful mistrust of government and health institutions by those most affected by the epidemic, and the determining influences exerted by its potential victims upon the entire societal response—these are new and contemporary phenomena.

Like other such modern, but noninfectious, epidemics as lung cancer and heart disease, AIDS depends upon voluntary and conscious behaviors. Thus the initial approaches to prevention involved educational attempts to persuade people to voluntarily modify their behavior.

Important features of the AIDS epidemic must be considered in order to understand the early perceptions by the most affected groups of what was happening around them.

First, the AIDS epidemic raced far ahead of medical recognition of its presence. Much of the infection that was to produce the epidemic in the United States had already occurred by the time the first cases of disease were recognized. This was especially true in New York City and San Francisco. The most rapid phase of transmission and infection in New York City, with respect both to gay men and intravenous drug users, took place in the mid to late 1970s, more than five years before we even knew the virus existed.

In some parts of the country, there has been a significant lag in both infection and the expression of HIV illness, compared to the high-prevalence cities exemplified by New York and San Francisco. But no corners of the country can remain entirely immune; seepage of the virus occurs through homosexual and heterosexual spread, drug use, and the now very rare (but still possible) contamination of blood and blood products. Low-prevalence areas have the most dramatic opportunities to enhance preventive efforts and reduce the eventual toll of AIDS, if the country learns the lessons that the virus has taught so far, and if we take full advantage of both education and public health control measures.

The evolution of the AIDS epidemic might be likened to time-lapse photography. Future events have been set in motion at a slow but persistent pace out of synchrony with usual human perception, and are playing themselves out in a relentless fashion. Infection itself is usually not noticed by the individual (because of the lack of immediate symptoms, or the presence of only a minor and protean illness several weeks after infection takes place). Then a long period of clinical latency intervenes, usually of several years, before definite symptoms appear. Even if at-risk individuals were to be repeatedly tested for antibody to the virus, six weeks or more would elapse between the actual date of infection and the appearance of a positive antibody test, with a small proportion of infected individuals remaining antibody negative for substantially longer periods.

In the early days of the epidemic, when the only recognizable benchmark of infection was the clinical diagnosis of AIDS, the cases reported were really "snapshots in time," taken approximately five years after the key events of infection. For example, the five men in Los Angeles who were the first people to be diagnosed in 1980 and 1981 with what later became known as AIDS had actually become infected back in the early to mid 1970s.

From the beginning, we played catch-up to an AIDS virus that had had a running start of five years or more. As we began to understand this fact, it became tragically clear that the most rapid phase of infection among urban homosexual men and among urban intravenous drug abusers was already over.

Working back from the numbers of AIDS cases diagnosed in any given year to the larger numbers of persons who must have been infected three to ten years previously, or from sample surveys, the best retrospective estimates show that the prevalence of infection among homosexual men and IV drug users moved very rapidly in New York City in the late 1970s and early 1980s.

This is not to suggest that effective efforts at preventing infection would have been unimportant in stemming the tide of the epidemic. On the contrary. Better prevention programs aimed at both homosexual men and intravenous drug users early in the epidemic would have resulted in a lower toll of illness and death over succeeding years, particularly among the women and infants infected in following waves of the epidemic.

No program or tool of prevention, however, would have deterred AIDS from its path to becoming an epidemic. A major modification of the epidemic among New York gay men and intravenous drug users could only have been made had successful prevention been designed and implemented well before 1982. It is difficult to see how that could have been possible, during a period when this virus was both unknown and unsuspected.

In areas of the country with low rates of infection, successful prevention efforts would have had a much greater relative impact through the 1980s, that is, the future rates of infection would have been kept lower. This also could have been true for high-prevalence cities like San Francisco and Los Angeles where the rate of spread of HIV among intravenous drug users was, and remains, much lower than in New York.

Especially in the early years after recognition of the gathering epidemic, before the advent of specific treatment, education and persuasion for behavioral change were the only reeds we had to lean upon, weak though they were. Recurrent themes throughout the first decade of the epidemic were the twin obstacles of inadequate efforts in marginally effective education, and resistance to the use of traditional measures of public health for control of the spread of

obstacles have allowed an increase in both the
and the length of its course yet to be run.
deal approach to dealing with outbreaks of in-
be summarized thus: an infection is recognized
of individuals; the appropriate transmission-
re put into place; no new cases occur during the
n interval of several days to a few weeks; the
and further spread aborted.

This was never a relevant model for AIDS. HIV infection was
widespread long before it was recognized; no truly effective trans-
mission-blocking measures existed and the rudimentary ones were
not used; the incubation period of HIV was years, not weeks, and
resulted in lifelong, not temporary, infectiousness. Silent transmission of the illness could, and did, occur for very extended periods.

But we could have done better, much better, by overcoming moralistic objections to widespread and explicit education regarding
dangerous sex and drug behaviors, and by employing vigorous public health measures to control the spread of the virus, especially as
the benefits of early diagnosis and treatment became evident.

Further, the virus initially expressed itself in the United States in
stigmatized groups—homosexuals and intravenous drug users, who
were the objects of strong social disapproval. Early media shorthand
like "the gay plague," or "the junkies' disease," allowed other people to distance themselves psychologically from the epidemic and
those directly affected by it. Most New Yorkers, and most Americans, viewed AIDS, until at least 1987, as somebody else's problem
—and a somebody for whom there was little concern or sympathy.

The most vicious yet telling expressions of this alienation were
comments frequently expressed in private settings about "AIDS as
the solution to the problems of homosexuality and drugs," or graffiti
such as the one I saw scrawled on a wall in Harlem in 1988: "When
will all the junkies die of AIDS and leave us in peace?"

Denial and alienation were enormous barriers to progress on the
first requirement for effective prevention: explicit awareness that a
problem exists.

This phenomenon of society distancing itself from a disfavored
group that is then blamed for causing an epidemic and endangering

others is not new. For example, during the nineteenth century, newly arrived immigrants to New York City were blamed for the cholera epidemics that swept the city in successive waves.

In Renaissance Europe, syphilis, which reached epidemic proportions after probable importation as a "new disease" from the New World, was at one and the same time referred to as the "English Disease," the "French Disease," and the "Spanish Pox"—always someone else's responsibility.

In the early AIDS epidemic, the larger society often acted as if the emergence of the virus was the "fault" of homosexual men and drug users—and as if AIDS would mostly be confined to them (with the exception of small numbers of "innocent victims" infected via blood transfusions or babies infected prenatally). It was when the fear of heterosexual transmission was perceived and even exaggerated, that the general public's concern for AIDS was activated.

In reality, of course, the HIVirus is, in its essential pursuit, a biological predator, no different from a trout or a hawk: it seeks out prey whose biological and social characteristics best mesh with its own.

Social and political changes were sweeping the world of homosexual men in the 1970s and early 1980s, especially in New York City and San Francisco. Those years saw the emergence of a visible gay community with strong social identity and expressiveness, and with significant political consciousness and power. The gay communities in New York and San Francisco were not only organized but educated and relatively wealthy, with well-developed formal and informal communications networks.

This visibly expressed community identity provided the base for the rapid political and health mobilization against AIDS by homosexual men.

It was the gay community itself that first came up with a set of responses to the epidemic. Those responses, which evolved along community action lines of the 1960s, are also symptomatic of AIDS' modernity, and will undoubtedly influence the way many other interest groups mobilize on other health issues in the future.

In the epidemic's earliest months, well before public health authorities offered specific recommendations for prevention, homosexuals debated heatedly among themselves about the extent to which self- or even government-imposed curbs on promiscuous sexual expression should be undertaken. This issue, which was to evolve into the struggle over the closing of the gay bathhouses in San Francisco and later New York, had symbolic as well as concrete power. Many homosexuals argued that any restraints on personal sexual liberty, whether self-organized or government-mandated, would be the first step in a repression of gay sexuality that would lead to reinstitution of sodomy laws and increased discrimination. Positions were taken all across the spectrum, from those who believed that free and unlimited expressions of sexual individuality were so central to gay identity that any restrictions would destroy that identity, to others who saw the primacy of the threat of rapidly spreading fatal infection.

The earliest mobilization by homosexuals in response to the epidemic came even before it was clear what the nature of the disease was, or what its cause or modes of spread might be. Gay men were ill and dying and the earliest voices of warning, such as that of New York playwright Larry Kramer, were loud in their claims that medicine, science, and government were criminally ignoring the growing problem, and that the gay community had to organize not only for its own defense, but also to force an adequate response from the rest of society.

The gay community's organized response to the epidemic evolved through four stages: the development of community-based self-help and advocacy organizations such as the Gay Men's Health Crisis; the evolution of broader advocacy, lobbying, and funding organizations such as the American Foundation for AIDS Research; the formation of effective Washington lobbying arms; and the rise of militant activism as exemplified by the radical tactics of ACT-UP (AIDS Coalition to Unleash Power).

This was, as we shall see, an intensely political set of reactions. Therein lies an important fact that is basic to an understanding of the history of the epidemic: it was, from the start, defined in political terms, especially by the gay community. This political aura—increasingly an aura of strident conflict—permeated all thought, action, and response to the epidemic.

Homosexual men in New York City, as elsewhere, were struggling for political status and recognition. A gay rights bill had been introduced six times by Mayor Edward Koch, beginning in 1978, and was vetoed five times by the City Council. It was finally passed by the Council in 1986. Political expression and protection of individual rights were of utmost concern to the gay community, and the threat of AIDS was placed squarely in that context.

But homosexual organizations and individuals also were ambivalent about AIDS as a mobilizing issue. Having experienced discrimination, many gays feared AIDS would lead to heightened homophobia, aversion, and overt repression. Some saw AIDS as a threat to hard-won civil rights, especially in the early days when the communicability of the virus was exaggerated and there were calls for mass quarantine. The media carried many accounts of discrimination against persons with AIDS, as well as against homosexual men who were perceived (for the most part inaccurately) as presenting a risk of infection to others: the waiter in the restaurant, the instructor at the aerobics studio, the neighbor in the apartment upstairs.

Society at large was slow to accept that HIV could not be transmitted by casual contact, especially since physicians and scientists were reluctant to make absolute statements concerning safety and talked only of probabilities. The public wanted the certainty of assurances, and was impatient and distrusting of scientific phraseology that was widely regarded as hair-splitting, equivocating, or both. As a plague of mysterious origins but associated with highly personal behavior, AIDS played easily into magical and taboo-laden concepts of "uncleanliness."

Conservatives and right-wing ideologues often proposed extreme measures for isolating those presumed to be infected. In 1985, for example, William Buckley published an op-ed piece in the *New York Times* in which he proposed tattooing infected homosexuals and drug users, the latter on the arm and the former on the buttocks, as a measure to contain the virus. Especially early in the epidemic, when the cause of AIDS and the routes of transmission were less clear, there were countless incidents of discrimination: loss of jobs and housing, shunning by friends, colleagues and relatives, refusal of transport by ambulances, refusal of dental and medical care, refusal by undertakers and funeral homes to handle bodies, and many others.

As the effects of discrimination mounted, AIDS became even more politicized, and more and more an ambivalent concern within the gay community. Beneath their essential truths, slogans such as "AIDS is not a gay disease" and "AIDS does not discriminate" illustrated the poignancy of this ambivalence. On the one hand, the gay community wanted to convey the urgency of the threat and to goad a reluctant and often hostile society into action. On the other hand, calling too much attention to the concentration of HIV infection among homosexuals and bisexuals carried other threats. These concerns were particularly acute for many closeted homosexual and bisexual men.

A fabric of language more related to politics than to reality grew out of this ambivalence. When combined with intense media involvement, the epidemic became almost as driven by popular misperception, on all sides, as those epidemics of former centuries. Similarly, the psychological power of blame (divine or otherwise), impurity, and retribution for violation of taboos was immense, and directed by the majority society at homosexuals and drug addicts.

There was, and remains, a reservoir of rage among gay men about the epidemic. The physical horrors, the decimation of friends, and the hostility of the larger society all seemed especially cruel coming just as political and social barriers against homosexuals had seemed to be easing. It is perhaps not surprising that prominent among gay perceptions was the idea that heterosexual institutions were, deliberately, doing far less than their best to respond to the epidemic among gays. This formulation had enough reality mixed into it to keep it vibrant and growing, and it was to be increasingly reflected in the radical stance of gay advocacy organizations.

There arose another deeper ambivalence among homosexuals. On the one hand, many stressed that this was not "the gay plague." AIDS and homosexuality were not synonymous. Yet the epidemic was so pervasive in gay life that in a strange way it cried out for ownership: "only we can really understand this; only we can really define this; this is ours."

The pain of this ambivalence—defining oneself by the dimensions of a great external threat or injury—is not confined to this epidemic. It is a common experience of minority racial and ethnic groups and oppressed political and religious bodies.

The 1970s and early 1980s had seen an explosion of gay sexuality accompanying the gay rights movement and the "uncloseting" of large numbers of homosexual men, especially in cities with a history of relative tolerance. In these sexual magnet cities, overt expressions of gay sexuality flourished. By their own reports, many men had large numbers of sexual partners annually, often numbering in the hundreds and even in the thousands. Frenetic casual and anonymous sex was widespread among homosexual and bisexual men. Bathhouses, back rooms of bars and clubs, and other public settings such as erotic bookstores and movie theaters were, in effect, wide open. Sexual practices such as anonymous group sex, sado-masochistic fantasies enacted with physical trauma, penetration of rectal orifices with penises, fists, and blunt objects—all these practices and more were accompanied by extremely high rates of sexually transmitted diseases and set the scene for the rapid transmission of HIV once it appeared in the late 1970s. Rates of rectal and oral gonorrhea in males soared.

Another indicator of high rates of sexually transmitted diseases among gay men is that during the 1970s almost 90 percent of all reported cases of syphilis in New York City were among males. Such a large male-female discrepancy in this disease would not be expected among a heterosexual population. In the later 1980s, as homosexual men reduced high-risk behavior and as the crack epidemic caused syphilis to increase rapidly among women, this ratio reversed, and slightly more new syphilis cases were reported among females than among males.

The unrestrained sexuality and promiscuous behavior of large numbers of homosexual men in New York and San Francisco was, in fact, the single most important and necessary element accounting for the nature of the AIDS epidemic among this group, just as was the practice of sharing injection equipment among intravenous drug users. The bathhouse/sex club and the drug shooting gallery were the equivalent seedbeds of an explosive epidemic. In both instances, large numbers of people engaged in very high risk behavior repeatedly, and often anonymously.

Without those institutions AIDS would still have existed and the HIV infection would still have spread, but the epidemic would have proceeded at a much slower pace and with much less intensity.

The high visibility and fears—both real and imagined—surrounding AIDS spurred gay community action. But there were serious conflicts, many of which remain to this date, between the realities of risk, infection and prevention, and the way people wished to perceive these issues. Tremendous obstacles to education and effective public health action were thrown up by the desires of the gay community to see things the way it wished them to be, rather than the way they were. The politics of that gap between desire and reality explains much of the strength of the more radical gay AIDS organizations that were to arise in the later 1980s.

A 1989 National Research Council study on AIDS notes that "before the viral cause of AIDS was known or detectable, behavioral research had shown that being sick with AIDS or showing laboratory signs of immune deficiency was associated with (1) a large number of different sexual partners; (2) receptive anal intercourse or other rectal trauma; (3) the use of bathhouses for sexual contact; (4) frequent infection with sexually transmitted diseases, particularly gonorrhea, syphilis, and enteric parasites; (5) sexual contact with gay male residents of New York City; and (6) the use of inhaled nitrites." Both before and since the discovery of HIV, the advocacy groups, particularly gay advocates, have often resisted moving or even speaking about ways to approach these issues directly.

More than with any other health issue, an entire semantic orthodoxy has grown up around AIDS. Much of it is politically driven AIDSpeak, and most of it relates to issues of concern to gay men. For example, this orthodoxy frowns upon describing "high-risk groups," but rather prescribes reference to "high-risk behavior." There are no "AIDS victims," but rather "Persons With AIDS (PWAs)." Referring to babies with AIDS as "innocent victims" is forbidden because that implies that some other victims are "less than innocent" and thus presumably "guilty." One treads lightly with "partner notification" rather than "contact tracing" of people who are or were sex or needle partners of those with AIDS, and thus might benefit from knowledge of their own possible infection plus ability to infect others. Shibboleths and half-truths such as "Education is our only weapon against AIDS," and "Confidential testing and partner notification drive people away from AIDS testing," which are based on little open constructive debate and even less upon any data, risk becoming self-fulfilling prophecies.

At a scientific meeting in New York City in 1988, Dr. David Rogers, an eminent senior medical figure who has served on virtually every New York City, New York State, and Presidential AIDS Commission, was loudly booed and hissed by gay members of the audience when, in describing the origins of the epidemic, he referred to "promiscuous homosexual behavior." Dr. Rogers had transgressed AIDSpeak boundaries.

These Orwellian semantics are destructive in their restrictive effects upon thought and action, diversionary in the considerable amount of energy that is wasted upon them, and also indicative of how, as we shall see below, the politics of AIDS too often gets in the way of effectively meeting the challenges of the epidemic.

## Infection Versus Civil Rights

All significant public health issues have important social and political parameters, but AIDS was the first major public health crisis in modern times in which the social and political parameters were defined, indeed set, before the relevant scientific underpinning was understood. That made an enormous difference, and one that often worked in opposition to the control of the epidemic. The social policy concerning AIDS has consistently been in advance of, and not guided by, the biomedical knowledge that should have informed it.

The initial public policy responses to the epidemic were designed as if the most important criterion was to protect civil liberties from abuse by public health actions. Thus, rather than searching for the most powerful disease prevention strategies compatible with the protection of individual rights, the conventional wisdom in AIDS policy became a watered-down version of the opposite: a civil rights strategy against which public health actions were to be measured. This was especially true in New York and California, where gay advocacy groups exerted political leverage in response to the epidemic.

It was this context that led to the long delays in closing gay bathhouses in San Francisco and New York, and to the many constraints to the widespread use of the antibody test, even under conditions of confidentiality, consent, and counseling. Concerns of the gay advocates were based, of course, on real experience with discrimination, directed against homosexuals in general and reaching new heights during the AIDS epidemic.

The ultimate fear of gay advocates was that panic might lead to widespread discrimination in housing, employment, and health care against anyone perceived to be homosexual and, beyond that, to mandatory testing, the compiling of lists of infected persons for various purposes of control, and mass quarantine of the infected. Indeed, any reading of history would have to acknowledge that the resort to such measures, though highly unlikely, was not impossible.

It was this set of concerns that led to the advocates' strong resistance to two methods of public health control of infectious diseases, especially diseases that are sexually transmissible: contact tracing (partner notification) and mandatory reporting of the names of infected individuals to public health authorities. These traditional measures of disease control were, in fact, blacklisted from AIDS prevention efforts in the early years of the epidemic.

My own views on the balance between public health control measures and protecting civil liberties had been evolving and changing since 1986. Like most of my public health colleagues, I had begun with a sense that because we were unable to offer effective medical intervention for HIV infection, and because the existing balance between public anxiety and active discrimination was delicate, we should avoid mandatory reporting, keep testing anonymous, and put the bulk of our prevention efforts into education and counseling.

But the evolution of the epidemic increasingly convinced me that those initial views had to evolve with it. The epidemic's shift toward minorities, drug users, and heterosexual transmission meant that risky behavior became increasingly difficult to identify in any given individual, and that risk-reduction education was ineffective. Our inability to track the virus's progress closely and to demonstrate that we could get ahead of the spread of HIV with preventive efforts was painfully evident.

These frustrations made the use of traditional public health measures more appealing, and I came to believe that they could be implemented with due protection of individual rights. Surely it must be possible to strike an appropriate balance between protecting the public health and protecting civil liberties, yet we were not allowing ourselves adequate scope for the former. Our ability to use the antibody test in New York was minimal relative to the need; our mandatory reporting system (but reporting of cases of AIDS, not of asymptomatic people infected with the HIVirus) was working but giving us information five years out of date. The fledgling partner notification program we began in 1987 was anathema to most AIDS advocates and even resisted by some of our own Health Department staff.

We were falling further and further behind the virus. A few low-prevalence states, notably Colorado under the leadership of Dr. Thomas Vernon, its Health Commissioner, were demonstrating that it was possible to implement a program of HIV reporting and vigorous contact tracing while preserving confidentiality and offering the option of anonymous testing. By mid-1987, I was convinced that if we were to have a chance of building an effective prevention program where it counted most—in the high-prevalence localities—we had to move in the same direction.

But what pushed my thinking in these directions most strongly was the emergence of hope in therapy. By 1987, early identification of infection was in the clear best interests not only of society but of the individual. How could we ignore the rights of individuals at risk who were, increasingly, minority women often unaware of their specific risk? I felt strongly that they had a right to know their risk and status as well as the steps that they might take to protect themselves or to seek medical management for HIV infection as early as possible.

We could and did increase our anonymous test sites as rapidly as possible and expand confidential testing in hospitals and doctors' offices to the limits of our influence. But what was needed was contact tracing and mandatory infection reporting—the very things most opposed by the AIDS advocacy groups.

To move toward more of a public health approach to the epidemic and to marshal the public support to do so, two preceding issues had to be addressed: creating a rational public view of the dynamics of HIV transmission, and providing a legal bulwark of confidentiality and antidiscrimination.

My main strategy for fostering a rational public view of the risks and realities of the epidemic lay in using all available opportunities for frank and explicit discussion.

In October 1985, the New York State Public Health Council had issued emergency regulations aimed at curbing high-risk sexual activity that led to the spread of HIV. These regulations had been the basis for closing the bathhouses and sex clubs in New York City. But in their definition, the Public Health Council listed only anal intercourse and fellatio as high-risk behaviors. I went before the council in November 1987 and asked that they revise the definition to take account of the undoubted risk in heterosexual penile-vaginal sex.

I had an additional objective in mind in that testimony. The City's Department of Consumer Affairs handled the inspection end of enforcing the state code's regulations governing unsanitary commercial facilities. Since October 1985, many types of commercial arenas of on-premises sex had been inspected. There were eighty-five of these commercial establishments inspected in all, most on multiple occasions. Four establishments were closed, based upon evidence that demonstrated that high-risk sexual activity occurred on a continuous and regular basis, condoned by management. These establishments included two gay bathhouses, a heterosexual swingers' club, and an S&M bar. Other establishments closed voluntarily.

After the initial closings, the gay bathhouses and sex clubs diminished in number or reduced high-risk activity. Undoubtedly this was at least as much due to the increasing awareness of the risks of unprotected anonymous sex as it was to the closings, but I believe both factors were important, and were interrelated. That this sort of activity continued could be demonstrated by the persistence of clandestine sex clubs, the use of bar back rooms for sexual activity, and the advertisements in printed publications of invitation to "private parties" and self-described orgies. These latter settings were clearly constitutionally protected, and the only antidote to the risk involved was public health education.

Sometime in early 1987, Angelo Aponte, the Commissioner of Consumer Affairs, asked whether I was interested in pursuing the commercial establishment issues further. His inspectors had gathered considerable evidence of widespread high-risk sex in a number of pornographic movie theaters. The inspectors were uncomfortable with this undercover work, and Angelo wanted to either have it go somewhere or to drop it.

I proposed that we meet with Doren Gopstein, the First Assistant Corporation Counsel, who had been in charge of the legal work for the bathhouse closings. We agreed that a great deal of high-risk sex was taking place in these theaters, and with the knowledge of management, and that it was appropriate to the public health to try to reduce or stop it. We also realized that, in the case of movie theaters, we would be in First Amendment territory that was much more difficult terrain than the bathhouses, the opposition on civil libertarian grounds would be stronger, and the prospects of withstanding court challenge might be lower.

Nevertheless, we resolved to press ahead, and adopted the following strategy: first, the Health Department would contact the four most flagrant of these theaters directly, warn them of the risks to public health, describe the actions that they should take to remedy these risks, and offer to work with them to achieve the remedies. In the meantime, the Consumer Affairs Department would continue its undercover inspections, and keep the Health and Law Departments briefed. If our educational approach succeeded, well and good. If it did not, we would be prepared to move legally to close one or more of the theaters, not only on the grounds of risk to public health, but also on the grounds of failure of lesser remedies. We discussed our plans with the Mayor, and had no difficulty obtaining his approval.

I wrote to the theaters, sent staff to work with them in defining risks and remedying them, and in general held out the carrot rather than the stick. I met with the Gay Men's Health Crisis, discussed what we were doing, and asked for their support in the educational effort. We continued this process until June 1988, when it became apparent that things were not improving.

Conditions were horrendous. The movie houses showed pornographic films to an almost entirely male clientele. Inside, theater seats, hallways, restrooms, and lounges were used for a wide variety of sexual acts, most between anonymous partners who cruised the theater. Mutual masturbation and oral sex was most common, but anal sex was also frequent. Often a single person would take on multiple anonymous partners. In short, the conditions were similar to those that had led to the closing of the bathhouses.

We resolved to go into court to force the worst theaters to close. Doren Gopstein, who would shoulder the burden of the legal argument, was a superb tactician and also a compulsive stickler for preparation and detail. Again and again we sent the inspectors in to ensure that our data was accurate and also current, and to anticipate and counter any arguments that our action was based on incomplete or misleading evidence.

Finally, in late September 1988, we went into State Supreme Court for a closure order. The police cleared and padlocked Cinema 14 on the East Side. There was much less protest from gay and civil rights advocates than I expected; perhaps the city was becoming aware of how tangible the realities of the epidemic were. Despite the appeals of Cinema 14's attorneys, the court upheld our closure request. We kept the theater shut down while we attempted to use that leverage to create improvement at the other theaters.

When continued inspections showed no changes at the other theaters, we went back to court in early February 1989, and got closure injunctions against two more theaters. (The fourth had decided to close on its own).

The *New York Times* noted:

> The closings drew criticism from advocates of gay rights and from a New York Civil Liberties Union official.
>
> Arthur N. Eisenberg, the Civil Liberties Union's staff counsel, said that because a theater is protected by free-expression provisions in the New York State Constitution, it cannot be closed for health reasons unless the city first takes lesser measures against the problem.
>
> "To the degree that they are closing down the entire enterprise because there are allegations of unsafe sex," Mr. Eisenberg said, "is that injunction too broad given that the rest of the theater is engaging in a First Amendment enterprise?"

The court once again sustained our argument; the ACLU blustered but did not go into court against us to challenge the order. None of the gay advocacy groups was pleased with the closures, but none challenged us legally, and the major organizations, Gay Men's Health Crisis and Lambda Legal Defense Fund, expressed their concerns in ambiguous terms. ACT-UP was, for once, silent.

About the only gay publication to try to whip up the issue was the *New York Native*, whose Editor John Hammond wrote:

> The Health Department's depositions against the theaters that were closed are virtually identical in tone and intent to depositions that were made against gay bars and brothels in the 1890's; only the excuse for the closings has changed: to promote sanitation rather than morality. . . . May I suggest that if he wants to contain the health crisis, Stephen Joseph should get off our backs, let our turf alone, fire his pecker checkers and instead hire educational teams to dispense information and condoms in places where sex occurs?

There was some small indication that the commercial establishments had gotten the message. Doren Gopstein was very tough in negotiating with the theaters, and we did not let them reopen until extensive changes in physical layout and operation were approved by us (in one case, the theater owner dropped the porno format). The courts upheld our positions without exception.

While it is fair to say that most gay New Yorkers were opposed to the actions, I had the sense that the opposition was largely based on fears of setting a precedent for gay repression. I received some of the usual hate mail, but I also received several anonymous letters from gay men describing their compulsive attraction to what they knew were life-threatening conditions in the theaters, and thanking us for closing them.

If only we could have also found a way to successfully move with police action to shut down the drug shooting galleries, I would have felt that we were taking a full range of responsible public health enforcement actions. But the Police Department told me repeatedly that this was impractical, that the galleries could just move from one abandoned building or apartment to another.

With the cinema closing strategy in process, we had been largely successful in eliminating high-risk sexual activity in open areas of commercial establishments. But some establishments had created a smaller space on the premises for the same activities. We found, for example, that some bathhouses hired people called "lifeguards" or "steerers" who, on seeing people engaging in high-risk sexual activities, would usher them into closed cubicles, and instruct them to keep the door closed.

I recommended amending New York State law to facilitate surveillance in nonlodging commercial establishments by authorizing the removal of doors or walls that prevented visible inspection. Such an amendment would have to be carefully designed so that its effect would be upon those commercial establishments that specifically provided closed-off areas for high-risk sexual activity.

This proposal raised issues for brothels and street prostitutes (both female and male); and sensitive First Amendment issues, such as in bookstores and theaters. These issues were difficult, but resolvable.

Unfortunately, no further legislative debate took place concerning where the lines of enforcement in commercial sex establishments ought to be drawn.

On the second issue—creating a shield of legal protection for the confidentiality of AIDS-related information—we had more success, though the process was, as usual, agonizingly slow. New York State and the city had strong antidiscrimination laws, and the city's Human Rights Commission was slowly establishing precedents of legal action regarding various forms of AIDS-related discrimination. The Mayor and Governor were strong and visible on this issue.

What was needed was a specific state law protecting the confidentiality of AIDS-related information, one that would enlarge public confidence in the use of the antibody test and reduce the likelihood of the use of information about a person's HIV status for repressive purposes.

By late 1986 I had begun working with the Health Department's General Counsel, Irwin Davison, on the drafting of such a law. We were hopeful that we could get mayoral endorsement and key legislative backing once we had a draft bill for negotiation and modification.

Our basic plan was for a two-pronged piece of legislation, one part protecting the confidentiality of AIDS-related information, and the second part specifying the limited circumstances in which the information could be used without consent.

But our initial effort was sidetracked. We found little support in either the clinical or political communities in 1986 for such legislation; most seemed to feel it was too touchy an area to maneuver in. We attempted to gain support from gay advocacy groups, but they were hostile to the limited disclosures idea and expressed concern that any confidentiality bill, no matter how well-intentioned or drafted, could be seized upon by conservative political forces and turned into a socially regressive piece of legislation.

Failing to get off the ground in 1987 only made us push harder for the 1988 legislative season, and by then the climate had changed. It was evident that the Reagan Administration was not going to help with federal protections. State legislative leaders became increasingly aware of the need for such a law, and we began to work closely with them and with the advocacy groups.

A joint State House and Senate AIDS Task Force hearing in October 1987 gave me an opportunity to launch a trial balloon. I argued that we desperately needed legislative guidelines for protecting the confidentiality of HIV information. Public assurance that the names of those participating in HIV antibody testing and their test results would be closely guarded would be the key to an effective voluntary testing program.

First, some people at risk of being infected and passing on the infection were not cooperating with prevention efforts because ordinary medical confidentiality was insufficient in protecting them from the discrimination surrounding AIDS. Indeed, the reporting of information in other public health programs, such as tuberculosis and sexually transmitted diseases, has historically been legislatively granted a higher degree of confidentiality. We needed a bill protecting AIDS information in the hands of doctors, hospitals, and other entities, not just in the hands of the Board of Health.

Second, the lengths to which the medical establishment has gone to maintain confidentiality has diverted resources from effective public health measures and testing facilities.

The questions following my testimony centered on the disclosure of HIV status, and I took the radical position that the physician has a duty to warn unsuspecting partners of an infected individual, a duty that is a professional and ethical obligation as well as good public health practice. This occasioned much debate, and the *New York Times* reported it this way:

> Proposing a sharp break from established policy and state regulation, New York City's top health official said yesterday that physicians and public health authorities should warn the sex partners of people infected with the AIDS virus of their substantial risk of infection.
>
> "There is no way we can force a patient to disclose the names of any persons," Dr. Stephen C. Joseph, the City Health Commissioner, said at a legislative hearing on AIDS. "However, in some circumstances," he said, "I believe a physician and a public health authority, acting as a physician, have the ethical obligation and moral duty to issue such a warning when

there is a clear risk of infection, even without the explicit consent of the patient."

Under current rules governing medical ethics and professional behavior in New York, physicians and hospitals are barred from breaching patient confidentiality. Violations carry civil penalties, professional sanctions, and possible lawsuits. . . . Dr. Joseph's proposal was described yesterday by legislators as a breakthrough in the public health debate over patient's rights and public health.

But state health authorities said they opposed such warnings [which] violated patient confidence and would undermine efforts to persuade people at high risk to seek medical counseling.

The *Times* went on to quote Mark Senak, director of legal services of the Gay Men's Health Crisis, who said that his group would not "categorically" oppose such warnings provided they were extremely limited and issued only when there was a clear risk of infection. Thomas B. Stoddard, executive director of the Lambda Legal Defense and Educational Fund, a gay rights organization, said his group opposed any breach of patient confidentiality, particularly in the case of AIDS patients. Exceptions could be made when "an AIDS patient wilfully refused to disclose his infection to an unsuspecting spouse." Stoddard said such warnings would apply mostly to heterosexual relationships in which one partner had no knowledge of the other's bisexual or "secret homosexual life style" or of intravenous drug use. Stoddard said there was no reason to warn homosexual partners, who, he told the *Times*, were fully aware of the risks involved.

My testimony represented a sharp departure from established public health policies dealing with AIDS, a classic case of civil rights conflicting with public health.

The *Times* also quoted my statement that if I had a patient infected with AIDS and the patient's wife did not know it, I would do everything possible to inform her.

From that point onward, and despite the differences of opinion on specific issues such as the duty to warn, there was a groundswell for an AIDS confidentiality bill. We garnered support from advocacy as well as medical organizations, and by the spring a bill based on our initial draft was working its way through the legislature.

Some compromises led to important modifications, however. The duty to warn provision was watered down into a "permission to warn" clause that indemnified the physician from liability if he chose to warn an unsuspecting partner at significant risk, after reaching a judgment that the patient would not disclose the risk to the partner. This weakened provision was virtually worthless in achieving the purpose.

We also lost the argument on the occupational exposure protections that we had wanted in the bill, by which police and public safety personnel who suffered an occupational exposure to an HIV-positive patient would be able to have the person's infection status disclosed to them.

This defeat was particularly galling to me, as I felt strongly that frontline emergency workers (the policeman who jabs himself on a concealed needle in the pocket of an apprehended drug suspect, or the emergency medical technician who jumps off the ambulance to give mouth-to-mouth resuscitation to a hemorrhaging accident victim) should have a special status granted them in return for their own risk-taking for the benefit of others. However, I was unable to prevail on this point with either the legislature or the city administration.

Beyond those two important deficiencies, the bill that emerged in the summer of 1988 was pretty much what we had wanted, though its implementation requirements were unnecessarily complex. The law gave New York State the strongest AIDS confidentiality protections in the nation, and strengthened my own resolve that the groundwork was laid for a more vigorous use of public health measures to contain the spread of the epidemic, and to protect the rights of individuals who were unknowingly at risk of infection with HIV.

Thus, the early perceptions of what this epidemic was were formed largely by the perspectives of the white, middle-class gay community, and most especially by new advocacy organizations that placed the issues firmly in a political context. Beginning with concerns that AIDS would bring increased stigmatization to homosexuals, it was a natural next step for them to define the controversies that surrounded AIDS as if they were primarily civil rights and civil liberties issues.

The HIVirus had chosen its hosts shrewdly. Yet even as it ravaged the gay community, it had found another set of hosts in quite a different community—intravenous drug users. Theirs would be a very different story. Lacking organized advocacy and living mostly in minority communities that sought to distance themselves as far as possible from AIDS issues, drug users played no significant part in the early political wars of the epidemic. They were, however, to pay the highest price for the false dichotomy that was set up in those earliest days: the dichotomy that held that strong public health action and protection of civil liberties were opposite and mutually exclusive courses of action.

# AIDS, Minority Communities, and Intravenous Drug Use

There are sections where the epidemiologists can go block by block in central Harlem and say, "This block will no longer exist in ten years because of AIDS." And the community-board leaders in Harlem are saying, "AIDS is not a problem for us. AIDS is a white man's disease."

—black social worker in Harlem, 1991

When will all the junkies die of AIDS and leave us in peace?

—Graffiti on a wall in Harlem, 1988

We are losing a generation.

—Margaret Heagarty, M.D., Chief of Pediatrics at
Harlem Hospital

CONSIDER THE MOMENTOUS IMPLICATIONS OF THE WIDESPREAD INFEC-tion of intravenous drug users with HIV. Here is a virus that pro-duces a lifelong infectious state, but which is silent for a period of years. In addition to the ability to infect others through the sharing of "works" (needles and syringes), the drug user is also able to infect his (or her) sexual partner and thus transmit the virus into the gen-eral population. Thus, the broadened base of HIV infection opened a silent channel for the heterosexual spread of the virus and the maintenance and further extension of the epidemic.

The channel was also silent politically. In contrast to the strong public expression and dramatic political action of homosexual groups, drug users are a silent underground. The illegality of intravenous drug use and its strong associations with other criminal behavior create a veil that is difficult to penetrate. The alienation of many addicts, the communication barriers inherent in the cultures of poverty within which many addicts live, and the mental illness associated with drug addiction have all led to obstacles inhibiting both analysis and responsive action.

Rather than representing a second wave of infection as was once thought, needle-sharing IV drug users were infected shortly after the virus arrived in New York, and the infection spread rapidly through those addicts who were most vulnerable—those who shared injection equipment with large numbers of people, especially in the shooting galleries of poor neighborhoods.

The direct injection of virus that is in the residual blood in a syringe is one of the most efficient ways known of transmitting HIV infection, second only to transfer via transfusion blood. (The transfusion recipient of a contaminated unit of blood has an 80–90 percent probability of being infected).

Since the probability of infection seems to be directly proportional to the amount of blood (and therefore to the quantity of virus) injected, the drug addict's practice of "booting," in which blood from the vein is repeatedly drawn back and forth within the syringe containing the drug that is being injected, greatly increases the chance of infection. Booting is used to wash the last traces of drug out of the syringe and into the vein, and is alleged by some addicts to produce a stronger rush. Drugs are more likely to be booted in poor neighborhoods, in situations where equipment is being shared, and thus where chances of one of the participants being HIV-infected are greatest.

HIV infection spread like wildfire through New York City's 200,000 heroin users, from 9 percent of infected intravenous drug users in 1978, to 38 percent by 1980, and to 50 percent or more by 1982. Again, as with homosexual men, the virus had ample time to seed this population long before AIDS was recognized. In addition, infection was transmitted from male IV drug users to their female partners, both through shared drug injection and sexual intercourse.

Of all New York women diagnosed with AIDS in the first five years of the epidemic, about two-thirds were infected through their own use of intravenous drugs, and about one-third through a sexual partner.

With such an efficient mechanism of transmission, not only did the virus spread rapidly in neighborhoods where drug use and poverty were concentrated, but the rate of spread intensified. If you were an uninfected heroin user visiting a shooting gallery in the South Bronx in 1978, and there were ten people "passing the spike," your chances of one of them being infected were less than 30 percent. By 1986, in the same situation, at least five of those other ten people would be infected, and your chances of escaping infection (in the unlikely event that, as a gallery frequenter in New York, you were still uninfected) would be close to zero if blood was transferred in the syringe passed to you.

Drug addicts are less visible than middle-class homosexuals to the surrounding society and to medical institutions. They are more susceptible to a wide variety of often fatal infections in their street life. It is likely that many cases of AIDS and AIDS deaths among drug addicts went unrecognized early in the epidemic, leaving the impression that the curve of infection among IV drug users lagged further behind that of gay men than it actually did.

However, it was recognized by 1986 that in high HIV-prevalence areas, drug addicts were dying at rates far in excess of former years. A series of studies carried out at the New York City Department of Health by Dr. Rand Stoneburner and his colleagues showed that while deaths from drug overdoses were constant over these years, deaths of drug addicts from a wide variety of infections, including tuberculosis, had skyrocketed. Similarly, in neighborhoods having a high prevalence of HIV infection, hospitalizations and deaths among young adults from pneumonias of all causes had increased manyfold.

Here was strong evidence that drug users, though less likely to be medically diagnosed with AIDS, were heavily infected with HIV, and were succumbing to a wide variety of infections.

Intravenous drug users are not a homogeneous population. Addicts are as diverse as the upscale Wall Street noontime user, the middle-class occasional weekend cocaine injector, and the three-bags-a-day gallery shooter. The rates of infection among well-to-do occasional heroin injectors who never share their equipment, or who only share works with a lover or spouse, are far lower than among the street addicts who frequent the shooting galleries. Unlike crack houses, shooting galleries are not generally places where drugs are sold. Rather, the gallery is a safe house where space and equipment for drug injection is available. In literal terms, the shooting gallery is where needles are rented and shared, and where HIV is a free add-on. In New York, a drug counselor who works with street addicts in one of the poorest areas of the city told me in 1988 that every one of her clients tested for HIV since 1986 was infected.

The social and economic parameters of needle sharing have led to significant differences in infection rates among addicts in various cities. The shooting gallery is mostly a phenomenon of impoverished urban areas in the Northeast, particularly New York and northern New Jersey, which have the highest rates of infection in IV drug users. In cities such as Los Angeles and San Francisco, where the shooting gallery is not an institution, infection rates among addicts are lower (though increasing). In cities such as Boston and Chicago, where the gallery pattern is intermediate, infection rates are probably somewhere in between the other two areas.

As AIDS cases began to appear among drug addicts, and as the needle connection became clear (in 1982 and 1983 in New York), the word on the street must have spread rapidly that a new deadly disease was killing junkies. Nonetheless, very little behavior changed in response.

With no political standing, with no existing community organization, and with even greater social disapproval than beset homosexuals, the "invisible community" of drug users probably saw the onslaught of the AIDS epidemic as just one more high-risk hazard in a life already fraught with risks. Indeed, early in the epidemic, to many addicts AIDS may have seemed so remote a threat as to be virtually irrelevant compared with the short-term dangers of the street: the need to make a daily score, the risks of overdose or contaminated drugs, hepatitis, or blood poisoning.

The corollary danger, that of onward infection of sexual partners, was even less recognized. To some extent this was worsened by the regrettable slowness of public health authorities to emphasize the dangers of heterosexual transmission. Even after the shift, in 1987, to a new emphasis on the dangers of heterosexual transmission, there was little recognition by drug users of the dangers of heterosexual spread to their female partners. The consequences of this were to be enormous.

While the gay community saw AIDS as a direct threat to individuals and community alike, one that required political mobilization, IV drug users were preoccupied and far less organized. The early perceptions of minority communities regarding AIDS can be best characterized in one word: denial.

Black and Hispanic residents were very resistant to the idea that this growing epidemic had implications for them. Community, political, and religious leadership shrank from any association with the issue. Despite the rapidly growing evidence of the impact of AIDS on New York City's black community, not until late 1988 was a Black Leadership Commission on AIDS formed—and this in a city where blacks are intensely politically involved. As of this writing, no analogous organization with wide visibility in the Hispanic communities in New York exists.

Local community service organizations representing minority concerns about AIDS, and black and Hispanic individuals who spoke out and worked on AIDS issues, were few and far between. In February 1987, when the Federal Centers for Disease Control (CDC) convened a meeting in Atlanta to discuss AIDS and minority issues, Dr. Beny Prim, a black physician with long experience running drug treatment programs in New York City, became, I believe, the first person to call for minority professionals to take vigorous leadership in their own communities on AIDS issues.

Over the first five years of the epidemic, about half of AIDS cases in New York were among blacks or Hispanics, but 80 percent of cases in women were among blacks or Hispanics, and over 90 percent of children with AIDS had black or Hispanic mothers. The high rate of cases in minorities was similar in many other areas such as Florida, New Jersey, Texas, and the District of Columbia. Nationwide, the CDC's data also clearly reflected this fact. While less than 20 percent of the United States population, blacks and Hispanics accounted for 40 percent of the total AIDS cases, 70 percent of the cases among females, and 80 percent of the cases among children as early as 1986. The 40 percent of all cases occurring among minorities had been constant since 1984, when racial/ethnic breakdowns were first reported by public health authorities.

In San Francisco, however, the pattern was overwhelmingly one of white homosexual male transmission. Over the first four or five years of the epidemic, less than 15 percent of San Francisco's AIDS cases were among nonwhites, and less than 1 percent among females.

Because the early media image of the epidemic was so dominated by the San Francisco model of AIDS as a disease of white homosexuals and because the gay community organized effectively, a curious invisibility settled over the spread of HIV through inner city populations.

The CDC's earliest public health reports noted only in passing the disproportionate numbers of minorities among the drug-associated, female, and infant cases. Nowhere was there a clear statement of the future implications of disproportionate rates of AIDS among racial and ethnic minority groups. Perhaps bruised by the controversy over the labeling of Haitians as a high-risk group and the subsequent charges against it of racism, the CDC was reluctant to head into a situation with similar potential again.

But the CDC was not alone in avoiding focused attention to the obvious data. State and local public health authorities, the media, and the general public all ignored the apparent implications of the demographic data.

Unlike the pattern by which HIV spread among gay white men, the onward transmission in minority communities followed multiple routes, and the pool of those susceptible to new infection was not only large but also very diverse. More than one-third of black and Hispanic men with AIDS were infected via homosexual sex. Gay men have the potential to infect other homosexual men, women via bisexual activity, and both men and women by sharing contaminated drug injection equipment. Those men and women, in turn, have the potential for onward heterosexual transmission. Thus, with a small proportion of homosexual and bisexual infected men, but with a large number of intravenous drug users, minority communities had the potential that was greatly feared but which never materialized among white middle-class heterosexuals: a self-sustaining and growing epidemic, based largely on drug use, but increasingly on heterosexual transmission between unsuspecting partners, with additional fueling by the crack epidemic with its extensive sex-for-drugs transactions.

The initial surge of AIDS in the minority neighborhoods in New York City was dominated by the transmission of HIV among intravenous drug users, and onward from them to their sexual partners and unborn children. Because blacks constitute a disproportionate number of New York's heroin addicts, the rise of infection in black neighborhoods was rapid. By 1986, AIDS had become the number one cause of death among young black men and women, even though the HIV-related death rate among drug addicts was certainly underreported by as much as 50 percent. The situation was similar among Hispanics and only slightly less dramatic.

As women and newborn infants were diagnosed with AIDS in increasing numbers, the effects of the epidemic on minority communities became more visible. The "AIDS boarder babies," infants stranded for weeks or months in hospital wards because there was no place for them to go—some sick and dying with AIDS, some healthy but abandoned and awaiting increasingly scarce foster care placement—was the first stark fact that dramatized and brought to popular consciousness the toll that AIDS was taking on minority communities.

These children were under the care of the city's social service and welfare agency, the Human Resources Administration (HRA). The issue of their HIV status rose into sharp focus. Concern increased about whether the number of foster parents could keep up with the demand, especially as popular knowledge about the AIDS risks of these babies spread. In fact, HRA mounted a very successful, though limited, program to place HIV-infected babies with foster families. It was inspiring to meet these courageous foster parents, drawn from different classes and ethnic groups, who were full of love for these incurably ill children, and who asked for nothing for themselves but to give that love.

But were they representative of the much broader range of prospective foster parents? I argued that the city should allow a prospective foster parent to learn, on request, the HIV status of a child that was being considered for foster care or adoption. This position was supported by Bill Grinker, the HRA Administrator, but opposed by most AIDS advocates, and by many on our two staffs as well as staff members at the foster care voluntary agencies. They argued that the HIV testing of the babies was an intrusion into the rights of the biologic mother (who "might not want to know her status" or who might suffer the effects of discrimination if her status became known), and an intrusion into the rights of the child, leading to possible discrimination. I argued that in taking legal responsibility and custody, the city was responsible for the welfare of the child, and that early diagnosis would lead to better medical follow-up and general care (even if the HIV-positive infant turned out in the end to be carrying passive maternal antibodies and not be infected).

Further, I felt strongly that a prospective foster parent had a right to this important information, just as they had a right to other critical medical information concerning the child; it would be unfair and in no one's best interest to hide the information. If learning that the child was HIV-positive dissuaded the prospective foster parent, well it was better to have that happen than to have to deal with the consequences of "surprised knowledge" later when the child became critically ill—as one-third of the HIV-positive infants would.

Despite the opposition, Bill Grinker and I prevailed on this policy, gaining the Mayor's agreement. Our policy was not challenged in the courts; I'm not at all confident we would have won if it had been. The agencies reluctantly and slowly implemented the policy, which had taken almost two years from the earliest arguments to implementation.

The media began to cover the racial and ethnic dimensions of the epidemic, not so much the drug-related aspects of AIDS as the heterosexual transmission. I believe that the first newspaper feature article focusing upon race and AIDS did not appear until late 1986, written by Richard Goldstein in the *Village Voice*. From early 1987 on, a flood of media coverage connected heterosexual transmission among black and Hispanic New Yorkers with intravenous drug use.

# The Epidemiologic Shift

The great epidemiologic shift of AIDS from the gay into minority communities in New York City was neither absolute nor abrupt. Through the 1980s and into the early 1990s, the cumulative number of AIDS cases and deaths in homosexual men (including men of color) remained significantly greater than heterosexual and drug-related cases among minorities. The shift was a gradually rising trend line that represented an increasing share of the present, a dominant share of the future, and a changing public perception about the nature of the epidemic.

In New York, as HIV transmission rates among middle-class gay men fell (both as a result of behavioral change and of the saturation with infection of those at very high risk) beginning about 1986, and as new cases of AIDS in this group began to plateau, beginning as early as 1987, it became at last unmistakably evident that a major shift in the epidemic was in process. The watershed year in New York City was 1988, when for the first time new cases of AIDS among intravenous drug users exceeded the number of new cases among men having sex with men.

This shift had profound consequences. The most obvious was the changing racial and ethnic makeup of the patient population: the proportion of women and children among all AIDS cases steadily increased, making clear the true implications of heterosexually transmitted HIV infection in minority communities, as opposed to white middle-class fears for their own vulnerability.

The shift in the epidemic also had geographic consequences. No longer were the most intense foci of transmission in Greenwich Village and the West Side, but rather Harlem, Washington Heights, the Lower East Side, the black and Hispanic neighborhoods of

Brooklyn, the Bronx, and Queens. These were also the neighborhoods most heavily pressed by poverty and a host of other social
problems, and areas where health services were most strained.

Part of the shift to women was among prostitutes: IV drug use was
the major factor in the spread of the HIVirus to female prostitutes.
CDC studies in 1988 showed wide variation in rates of infection
among female prostitutes around the country—the key factor was
whether the woman was herself an intravenous drug user. This
could reflect either the woman's infection via the sharing of contaminated injection equipment, or her sexual infection via a drug-using
sexual partner who was himself infected as a needle sharer. In cities
such as New York where intravenous drug use among women is
closely correlated with prostitution, infection rates among prostitutes mounted rapidly, and reached 30 percent or more by the end
of the 1980s.

The connection between intravenous drug use and sex as transmission routes was also key in the entry of the virus into the city's
adolescent population. Adolescence, a time when many are experimenting with sex and drugs, provided for entry of the virus into the
general population, and again primarily in poor and minority areas.
By mid-1990, only 46 actual cases of AIDS had been diagnosed in
the city's adolescents, but several thousands of teenagers were infected and still without symptoms. In addition, a larger number of
AIDS cases diagnosed in people in their early twenties was the
result of infection undoubtedly acquired years before. Most worri-
some was that almost half of the diagnosed adolescents were females, far higher than the adult proportion of under 15 percent.
This suggested increased heterosexual transmission.

Many adolescents who experiment with intravenous drugs stop
before becoming continuous drug users. They are usually initiated
into drugs by an older addict with whom they are likely to share
injection equipment, in much the same way that a woman initiate
shares needle and syringe with her drug-using male sex partner.
Even if the teenager stops drugs shortly, the chance of infection in a
city like New York, where most adult intravenous users are already
infected, is very high. The infected teen, who probably does not
regard himself as an intravenous drug user, is then infectious to all

future sex partners who, in many cases, have no way of knowing about this drug-using past. The virus can circulate rapidly through an adolescent population in which traditional risk behavior is hidden.

A tragic anecdote illustrates this point. Identical male twins, raised in New York City, were members of a rock band in the late 1970s, and very briefly used heroin together. They moved to Florida in the 1980s. The young men had stopped and "forgotten" their drug use. Both married, in their mid-twenties, and fathered children. It was only when the infant of twin A was diagnosed with AIDS that it was discovered that both adult twins, their wives, and one child were HIV-infected.

A particularly vulnerable group of adolescents in this regard are the runaway, "throwaway," street kids, who number in the tens of thousands in New York City. Many use drugs heavily, and many engage in prostitution to survive. The young boys are frequently involved in homosexual prostitution, although often considering themselves heterosexual in their personal relationships (usually with girls who are themselves at very high risk, often being street kids and themselves prostitutes). In a 1988 joint study, the Health Department and Covenant House found that 8 percent of Covenant's adolescents were infected. The difference between male and female rates was negligible—9 percent in males, 7 percent in females.

Further, the epidemiologic shift began to put extreme pressures on an already stressed system of public sector services. Despite a return to more general prosperity after the fiscal crisis of the 1970s, social services in New York were unable to cope with a rising tide of homelessness, scarce medical care, deinstitutionalized mentally ill people, and the violence and social destruction of the drug epidemic.

By the late 1980s, AIDS, though not the major factor in the gridlock in hospital emergency rooms, was rapidly becoming the additional burden that might break the back of the public hospitals. Social services, particularly those related to children, the homebound ill, and the shelter of the homeless were all pushed to the brink by the pressures of HIV infection among minority New Yorkers.

# Denial in Minority Communities

In contrast to the response of the gay communities, the minority communities in cities did not rally quickly to defend themselves against the epidemic, nor did they demand (or receive) help from government or private institutions. Where many gay men had access to private physicians who early on developed expertise in recognizing and dealing with HIV-related illness, most minority patients lived in communities pressed by other severe health and social problems, including the inability to pay for health care.

Further, the intravenous drug user, gateway to infection in poor neighborhoods, was much more resistant to warnings. His sexual partner was likely to be unaware of her actual risk and therefore unable to protect herself by negotiating safer sex, despite the efforts of public health agencies to provide this information. (Some 90 percent of infected IV drug users were male, thus the transmission pattern tended to be male-to-female or male-to-male.)

Had they been implemented vigorously, traditional public health approaches might well have slowed the further spread of infection among women in minority communities. But the political and social context was already set, molded by the gay community's strong resistance to the widespread use of the antibody test and their determined opposition to mandatory reporting and voluntary contact tracing. This resistance crippled the use of these public health tools in New York and elsewhere, and also augmented minority resistance to the concepts. ("Well, you didn't use these methods as long as it was the white gay community, but now that it's a question of blacks and Hispanics, you want to call out the Health Police.")

We shall return in later chapters to a more detailed discussion of the debates over testing, reporting, and contact tracing. The important point for the moment is that no techniques—neither community self-action, nor effective public health education, nor public health disease control measures—were brought to bear on the early spread of HIV within minority communities.

Given the connection with intravenous drug use, the epidemiologic shift of HIV into poor, minority, drug-ridden neighborhoods by the late 1980s was inevitable.

Because of the close associations with homosexuality, which black culture condemns, and drug addiction, from which black communities carry the greatest burden, black political and media personalities wanted to distance themselves from the epidemic. I remember a hearing in which I attempted to impart a sense of the seriousness of the epidemic to the black and Hispanic caucus of the New York City Council. My assertions that our data showed that 30 percent of black men and 40 percent of Hispanic men with AIDS in New York City were infected by sex with another man were met with stony silence and no follow-up questions.

The black clergy, the most important and influential conservative force in the community, were especially late in mobilizing their congregations against the epidemic. Strongly held perceptions of homosexuality as sin, and great difficulties in speaking to their congregations in the explicit and graphic terms about sexuality that were inherent in the epidemic, left black clergy virtually absent from any early role, apart from vague exhortations to abstinence from sinful behavior.

Frank discussions about racial characteristics of the epidemic were often perceived by blacks as racist. I spent a very uncomfortable half-hour before a live, middle-class black television audience while taping "Tony Brown's Journal." The host accused me of spreading a racist doctrine because I insisted that black women in New York City were at risk of AIDS—the percentage of HIV-positive infants born to black mothers in the city was severalfold that of infants born to white mothers. Brown was adamant that what should be said was that black women who have sex with IV drug users were at risk. My response that women didn't always know the drug histories of their current or former partners cut absolutely no ice with either host or audience. (Currently, in the city's poorest and most heavily infected neighborhoods, all of which are overwhelmingly minority, the prevalence of HIV infection among women of reproductive age is as high as 5 to 10 percent, an enormous figure in public health terms.)

The sensitivity of the black community to possible racial implications in the AIDS debate was heightened by deep suspicions of the government's concerns for minority health problems. In fact, the severe nature of these problems—the inaccessibility of health services, infant mortality, the lack of prenatal care, and above all, the ravages of the drug epidemic—helped to diminish the importance of focusing upon AIDS as a health priority for blacks.

The scars left by the Tuskegee experiment—in which United States Public Health Service physicians allowed black men with chronic syphilis to go without penicillin treatment for decades as part of a controlled study of the effects of such treatment and long after the medical benefits of penicillin in treating syphilis were clearly established—run deep in black consciousness. Memory of Tuskegee (the experiment did not end until 1972) not only exacerbated suspicion of government proposals for action, but also fueled a conspiratorial theory among blacks that AIDS resulted from a biological experiment, gone awry, performed on Africans by the United States government. As we shall see in discussing proposals for needle exchange, charges of genocide arise quickly in many controversial health policy debates concerning the black community.

A similar denial occurred in the Hispanic community, where the aversion to open recognition of homosexuality and bisexuality is even stronger, and the reluctance to explicitly discuss drug addiction is similar. Hispanic political figures were even less willing to be identified with AIDS issues than their black counterparts. The diverse Hispanic communities—based on different countries of origin, and with different values, rates of drug abuse, and even divergent dialects—have far less political cohesiveness and organizational strength than blacks. Thus Hispanics had less ability to respond as a community to the epidemic, particularly as the Hispanic media tended to duck explicit discussions of sexuality, especially concerning the empowerment of women to protect themselves from infection.

The results were grim. With roughly equal black and Hispanic populations in New York City, there were far more cases of AIDS among black women (1,703) than among Hispanic women (1,051) by 1989. But if those women infected by their own drug use are eliminated and only women infected by sexual contact are counted, more Hispanic (346) than black women (332) were infected by 1989.

As the dominant religious force among Hispanics, the Catholic Church played a complex role. The Archdiocese of New York took an early and active major part in caring for and developing services for people with AIDS. But the Church's vocal condemnation of homosexuality, its strong opposition to condom promotion, its insistence that the only legitimate prevention of sexual infection lay in abstinence, and its unwillingness to condone explicit education—all exacerbated the unfortunate denial of the epidemic among Hispanics.

At the end of the first decade of AIDS, Hispanic communities in New York and in most of the rest of the country still did not possess a clear and organized sense of the relevance of the AIDS epidemic to them.

# 5

## Heterosexual Transmission, Realities and Fantasies: The Panic of '87

AIDS is now running rampant.

—Masters, Johnson, and Kolodny, summarizing their view that AIDS had moved into the general heterosexual population in *Crisis: Heterosexual Behavior in the Age of AIDS*

Now we're gonna have the daylights scared out of us unnecessarily. But I would say, "Don't let AIDS ruin your life."

—Helen Gurley Brown, editor-in-chief, *Cosmopolitan*

DURING THE EARLY YEARS OF THE EPIDEMIC, THE PUBLIC THOUGHT OF AIDS as an epidemic largely confined to white gay men. This was true not only in San Francisco, where more than 90 percent of cases were indeed among homosexual men, not only among the gay advocacy groups that were so effective in mounting community-based self-education campaigns, not only among the media, but even in those cities like New York, where the plight of intravenous drug users should have served as a warning signpost to the future. Perhaps only in northern New Jersey, where the large majority of cases were recognized to be among poor minority people was there a frank recognition of the course the epidemic would eventually take. But the example of New Jersey had little effect on the overall conception of the nature of the epidemic.

The data from which correct inference could have been drawn

were available from the early weekly reports of the CDC, beginning in 1982, but there was a general disinclination to analyze the data for an accurate prediction of the future.

## First Problem: Denial by Public Health

The epidemiologists of the New York City and State Departments of Health, who were tracking and recording almost 40 percent of all the national cases in the first four or five years of the epidemic, demonstrated strong (and, to me, inexplicable) resistance to any focus on the possibility of significant heterosexual transmission of the virus. When I assumed my post as Health Commissioner of New York City in May 1986, one of my senior staff proclaimed to me at our first meeting: "There is no evidence that heterosexual transmission occurs in North America."

The New York City Department of Health's sophisticated surveillance methodology, which assigned a risk factor to each reported case of AIDS, was attempting to discover the pattern of the virus's distribution in the population.

Validation studies from hospital records and death certificates indicated that physicians in the city were actually reporting some 85–90 percent of all cases of AIDS that they saw, a phenomenal percentage compared to other reportable diseases, where the index of reporting is often only 10–30 percent. The assignment in a given case of the risk factor(s), such as men having sex with men, or intravenous drug use, were derived either from the reporting physician's statement or from an interview with the patient by our staff. Our interviewers rapidly became skillful in assessing a person's risk behavior, despite the sensitive and often uncomfortable nature of the material discussed. By 1985, those cases in which the department was not confident enough to assign a specific risk factor amounted to less than 2 percent of all reported cases in the city, compared to almost 7 percent of cases nationwide.

Of course, there were possible sources of error in the risk assessment procedure and in the system of classifying risk for analysis of the overall pattern of the epidemic. But the major impediment to mapping the spread of the epidemic was that the data were based on cases of reported AIDS, not on the occurrence and patterns of HIV infection itself, since no widespread testing, let alone screening, was being done. Indeed, before the HIV antibody test became available in the spring of 1985, the only reliable way to survey the epidemic was to count diagnosed cases of AIDS. The importance of being sure that all surveyors were counting the same thing had led to a necessarily narrow clinical definition of reportable cases of AIDS, a definition that excluded various earlier stages and different forms of HIV illness (which did not meet CDC's formal AIDS definition) from the counts.

Women infected by a sexual partner, rather than by their own intravenous drug use, would have been expected on average to have been infected later in the epidemic than homosexual or bisexual men, or male intravenous drug users. Compared to men, fewer women would have had adequate time to become clinically ill with AIDS. Because these factors tended to undercount the actual number of women infected with HIV, the Department of Health should have been, in my view, more skeptical about what appeared to be a very small number of heterosexually infected women in the early statistics. Instead, the department continued to deny and downplay the future potential for heterosexual transmission.

Had larger samples of antibody test results been available earlier in the epidemic, this would have been clarified. But widespread resistance to the use of the antibody test had resulted in significant opportunities being lost for a timely understanding of the pattern of HIV infection. When, in 1988, we finally began to understand the extent of existing infection among women in New York City, the spread of infection was already much greater than was expected.

To deny the importance of heterosexual transmission, and especially infection of women, required a self-induced blindness to several existing patterns of HIV infection and its spread.

The first pattern involved the mechanics of transmission. HIV's major modes of transmission are by blood-to-blood transfer, sexual transmission, and "vertical transmission" from infected mother to fetus (either during intrauterine life or during the birth process).

The accumulated data from infected homosexual men showed that the greatest risk was in being the receptive partner in anal intercourse. Linking specific sexual behavior to specific levels of risk is of course very difficult scientifically. Many, perhaps most, sexual episodes involve more than one activity. Memory and interview techniques are far from infallible. The long latency period of HIV further complicates matters. But in the case of gay men, the role of rectal trauma seemed clear, and fit well with the blood-borne and semen-to-blood transmission hypotheses. What was much less certain—and remains unsettled to this day—was the extent to which other sexual practices (oral-genital, oral-anal) involved any risk of HIV transmission.

The question immediately arose, therefore, whether there was something specific in male-male transfer of semen to blood, or whether male-female or female-male transmission could also occur. In theory, there seemed no good reason why this could not be the case. It made good intuitive sense to conclude that the ring of superficial blood vessels in the anus and rectum might be more easily traumatized, but that microscopic bleeding in the vagina during intercourse, or semen flooding an abraded surface of the uterus around the time of menstruation, would also fit the evolving model of transmission. In fact, the relative risks of these hypotheses fit quite neatly with the data: the largest number of sexually transmitted cases were among men having sex with men, the next largest were among females infected by a male sexual partner, and only a very few cases were among men infected by a female sexual partner.

Though admittedly theoretical, the models of transmission should have suggested a strong hypothesis that HIV could be transmitted heterosexually as well as between men, until proven otherwise. Unfortunately, the New York City Department of Health took the opposite view until 1986. Again, much early opportunity for education and prevention was lost.

Despite the Department of Health's position, considerable evidence pointed toward heterosexual transmission. From the earliest recognition of the epidemic in Africa and Haiti, the prevailing mechanism of transmission was known to be heterosexual. Various theories postulated reasons for more frequent heterosexual transmission in the Third World than in North America: very high prevalence of other sexually transmitted diseases that could assist HIV transmission, poor hygiene and more frequent genital lesions, and a low rate of male circumcision: all these factors were proposed as ones that could facilitate female-to-male, and male-to-female transmission.

But the rapid spread of HIV infection in both sexes in Africa and Haiti certainly should have put the burden of proof on those who wished to deny the possibility of heterosexual transmission in the United States. And certainly by late 1985, studies pointing to heterosexual transmission, done in a number of American cities as well as in New York itself, should have established not only the danger but the present reality of heterosexual transmission—and especially the infection of women.

The epidemiology of AIDS over the first decade of the epidemic consistently reflected three important points with respect to heterosexual transmission and the infection of women and children with the HIVirus. First, the proportion of New York City females with AIDS compared with males began at a ratio of only about 1 to 13. By the middle years of the decade, the ratio began to increase steadily to approximately double that early balance. A similar pattern was apparent nationally. Second, about two-thirds of New York City women diagnosed with AIDS were themselves intravenous drug users, and presumably infected by the use of contaminated injection equipment—with an important caveat, as follows:

Of those women presumed infected by a sexual partner, roughly 80 percent were infected by a male intravenous drug user, and about 20 percent by a bisexual man. Repeated studies have established that sexual contact with a drug user is by far the greatest sexual HIV-infection risk factor for women.

The question of transmission risks in female-to-female sexual activity has been repeatedly raised by gay and lesbian groups. Definitive data does not yet exist on this point. Clearly, there is theoretical justification for arguing that blood-to-blood exchange or vaginal fluid to blood exchange may occur during female-female sex. The vague but not disproven possibilities of infection via oral-genital or oral-anal sex also apply to female-female sexual activity.

But there is little or no scientific data to support high risks to lesbians. Of 7 cases of AIDS in New York City women who reported lesbian sexuality, all 7 also had a history of current or prior intravenous drug use, and/or of sexual relations with bisexual males or male intravenous drug users. This illustrates the difficulty of isolating one specific risk factor from among multiple risk behaviors. It is probable that the risk of lesbian HIV transmission is much lower than in other sexual activity. This interpretation led the New York City Department of Health and the CDC to forego listing female-female sex as a risk category in surveillance reports, despite the pressures from lesbian groups to do so. There is some truth in the argument that "if you don't look for it (i.e., classify it), you'll never find it." But a more serious consideration would be to avoid diluting the analysis of known high-risk factors in women: intravenous drug use and sexual contact with a male in one of the known risk groups.

It is important, however, that public health authorities continue to assess carefully the risk factors in women with AIDS who give a history of female-female sex. I certainly advise lesbian women to exercise the same caution over the (unproven) risks of oral sex, and to avoid rough sex play associated with bleeding as should heterosexuals and homosexual men, and to consider counseling and antibody testing for self and partner if there is any doubt about the noninfected status of both partners, especially given the common history among lesbians of past or current sexual relations with males (who may be bisexual, drug users, or heterosexually infected).

The third critical fact of heterosexual AIDS epidemiology is that heterosexual transmission seems to take place much more easily from male to female than from female to male. New York City through 1989 recorded only 8 cases of men (out of a total of almost 21,000) who were unequivocally infected by sexual transmission from a woman. By contrast, 793 women (out of 3,300 female cases of AIDS) or 24 percent of all cases in women, were judged to have resulted from sex with an HIV-infected man.

There was much argument during the 1980s about the reasons for this enormous disparity. The explanation generally favored by those who put less emphasis on heterosexual transmission is that the mechanics of HIV infection are directly responsible—that the virus moves more easily from semen through a damaged vaginal or rectal surface than from vaginal secretions through a male urethra or open penile lesion. This makes some intuitive sense, but no other sexually transmitted disease has such a dramatic discrepancy in the direction of infection. More important, in countries where the transmission of the virus has been overwhelmingly heterosexual, the sex ratios of males to females have been about equal. Several theories have been invoked to explain this, turning on a greater susceptibility to HIV infection of Africans as compared to North Americans because of hygiene and circumcision, and more frequent venereal infections, especially among those with open genital lesions.

An alternative argument is that far from there being something different about the amount and direction of heterosexual transmission of HIV in Africa from the United States, there is something wrong with the way the North American data are collected—undercounting heterosexual transmission in general and female-to-male transmission in particular. This line of argument was widely adopted by those who criticized the New York City Department of Health in the early years of the epidemic for downplaying heterosexual spread of AIDS.

Over 2,000 New York City women through 1989 were labeled as being infected because of their own intravenous drug use, a number over two and a half times higher than the women considered to have been infected by sex with a man at risk. But many of those drug-using women were also sex partners of men who use intravenous drugs. How can the scientist be sure that the actual mode of infection in any given woman was from an infected needle in her own arm—and not sexual? There is no certainty, but in order to understand the flow of the epidemic risk must be assigned somewhere, to a single factor in most cases. Being an intravenous drug user takes priority over any other known or unknown risk. Thus a female drug addict is categorized as infected via her own drug addiction. Bloodstream injection is far more efficient than sexual transmission.

Yet at some level this becomes a self-fulfilling prophecy. It is almost certain that some women listed in the drug risk category were actually infected sexually; what we don't know is how many, whether the numbers were large or small.

Clearly, the risk assessment and analysis method itself has inherent weaknesses that tend to undercount cases of heterosexual transmission—which is what the early critics of the city's methodology (which was, by the way, identical to that of the CDC) were pointing out.

When I arrived on the scene in 1986, I saw no feasible way to reformulate the surveillance methodology to solve this problem. Rather, the first priority was to emphasize clearly the major defined risk groups and behaviors. It was unrealistic in the extreme, however, to assume that no inadvertent erroneous categorizing had occurred. Such inaccuracies would have led to an underreporting of heterosexual transmission and risk. It seemed to me that the CDC-NYC practice of creating a separate category for men who carried both risks (sex with other men and intravenous drug use) showed clear recognition that a person's risk could not always be accurately attributed to a single factor. Rather than resisting the idea that heterosexual transmission was significant, health officials should have endorsed it. Many did.

Another possibility in assessing the large difference between heterosexual infection (particularly female-to-male transmission) in Africa and the United States is that this difference will decrease as time goes on. The later pattern in the United States of heterosexual transmission may tend more and more to approach the African pattern. Indeed, the proportion of heterosexually acquired AIDS cases in New York has been steadily increasing.

Even more striking is the pattern arising from the studies that have looked at infections among female prostitutes and the risk of their infecting male customers.

All early studies of female prostitutes in the United States showed clearly that rates of infection were most closely linked to intravenous drug use by the woman or by her frequent sexual partner(s). In other words, the chief risk factors for prostitutes, though greatly enhanced (in some of the urban areas studied, infection rates were as high as 30 percent), were similar to risks for other women.

All early studies also showed very low or nearly nonexistent risks of transmission from female prostitute to male customer. In part this may have been due to behavioral factors: prostitutes had markedly increased their condom use, and a significant fraction of their sexual encounters involve only oral sex. But these early studies did indicate that the risk of female-to-male transmission was very low, even among a population of women with high rates of infection.

Yet evidence shows that female-to-male transmission is increasing. While the city's Health Department found no evidence in 1987–88 for male infection from prostitutes, 1989 studies suggest that it may now be occurring. This may be a reflection of the rise in other sexually transmitted diseases among heterosexuals, making the HIV transmission patterns in New York increasingly similar to Africa. Open genital lesions facilitate the entry of the HIVirus, easing the path of heterosexual transmission, both male-to-female and female-to-male.

Even more disturbing was a study at a clinic in the Bronx in 1989, in which the Department of Health selected a group of men with a variety of venereal complaints but with no traditional risk factors for HIV infection. They had no history of sex with other men, or of intravenous drug use. They were, however, all heavy crack smokers. Among these men, the rate of HIV infection was 30 percent! HIV infection in sample surveys at the city's sexually transmitted disease clinics in 1988–89 were in the range of 7 percent for females and 9 percent for males, with rates rising to 19 percent in persons with open genital lesions. Similar rates were found in a study of homeless street adolescents who engage in prostitution and drug use, especially crack.

My own view is that we will indeed see an "African-like pattern" with regard to future heterosexual transmission of the virus in the United States, but that it will be mainly confined to specific geographic and demographic areas (that is, poor minority neighborhoods with many drug addicts) rather than spread across the city or nation.

A critical pattern in understanding heterosexual transmission is the racial and ethnic predominance of minority women and children who are infected. While 50 percent of all AIDS cases in New York City are among black or Hispanic people, over 80 percent of the city's female cases are among blacks and Hispanics, and 92 percent of the children with AIDS are black or Hispanic.

This disproportionate impact of infection on minority women and children is a direct result of the link between drug use and heterosexual transmission and has the most profound implications for the future of AIDS in the United States. But it also helps explain why, in the earliest years of the epidemic, heterosexual transmission was less visible than it should have been. Most of these HIV-infected minority women lived in very poor areas of the inner city, were themselves intravenous drug addicts or the partners of addicts, and were in only sporadic contact with the health system. Further, their own communities were engaged in a powerful denial of the relevance of the epidemic to blacks and Hispanics.

In 1988, the New York State Department of Health published a first survey of maternal infection. The results were startling. In New York City, one out of every 61 women giving birth was infected, compared to one out of 749 in the rest of the state. Within New York City, the prevalence of maternal infection was skewed toward areas of poverty and minority residents: for example, much higher in the Bronx than on Staten Island.

In late 1986 and early 1987, the perception of the heterosexual threat of AIDS began to swing to the other pole, and as with most such shifts, the threat moved from too little attention to exaggerated concern. Within a few short months, a strong wave of AIDS anxiety, fueled by the media, swept middle-class Americans, especially women.

To some extent it reflected catching up with the data, a gradual consciousness that HIV could indeed be transmitted heterosexually, and that such cases were being reported increasingly from within the United States. But this was not the whole explanation, because the incidence of AIDS among U.S. women was, from the very beginning, overwhelmingly among minority women; the wave of new anxiety was primarily among the white middle class.

By 1987, medical and public health AIDS experts were focusing increasing attention on heterosexual transmission, and those few who viewed it to be of little significance lost all credibility. In October 1986, the "Symposium on the Heterosexual Transmission of AIDS" was held at the New York Academy of Sciences under the sponsorship of Montefiore Hospital; in February 1987, a national conference on "Children, Adolescents, and Heterosexual Adults" was held in Atlanta, and in April of that year a "Surgeon General's Workshop on Children with HIV Infection and their Families" took place in Philadelphia. All three were meetings that involved most of the clinical and public health workers prominent in AIDS issues, and were widely reported in the press.

The public's growing awareness and concern over the rising numbers of AIDS babies also heightened the awareness of heterosexual infection. Almost 40 percent of these infants were in New York City, and another 15 percent in New Jersey. While these were overwhelmingly black and Hispanic infants whose mothers had usually been infected through intravenous drug use rather than sexual intercourse, the heavy focus of emotion and press attention on these children highlighted the message that "Women Can Get AIDS Too."

The death of Rock Hudson in 1985 is often described as a turning point in the nation's attitude toward the epidemic because of Hudson's star status and his role as a powerful and visible sex symbol to millions of white middle-class American women. The sudden revelation of his homosexuality and his death from AIDS evoked in women deep anxiety about the risk of contracting AIDS from a closeted bisexual man. In combination with growing scientific data, AIDS babies, and the increasingly shrill attention of the media to what was being billed as "the breakout of the epidemic into the general population," Rock Hudson's death had a powerful effect.

Public awareness of heterosexual transmission bypassed the real significance of heterosexual transmission: that heterosexual spread of HIV was concentrated in poor, drug-ridden communities. Concern focused instead on sensational news articles about individual middle-class white Americans who had "caught AIDS" by a transfu-

sion or blood-product-infected spouse, or from a past or current sex
partner who was a former drug addict or a bisexual man.

The debate became: will AIDS break out of the risk groups and
spread rapidly through middle-class America? Some argued, not
totally without logic, that AIDS had spread undetected in its first
waves and might do so again. The lack of a broad base of antibody
testing made it impossible to answer this question definitively at
first, although as a broader picture emerged in 1988 and 1989 from
military recruit studies, newborn anonymous testing in several
states, and results of voluntary testing, no evidence of a broad pattern of infection in nonminority women surfaced.

National newspapers and news magazines were crowded in early
1987 with stories of the feared breakout. Evening television news
was full of interviews such as the one in a bar in Snowbird, Utah,
crowded with affluent young skiers, who were being asked about
fear of AIDS and any consequent changes in sexual behavior. Much
was written, without much to base it on, about major changes in
American sexual mores, the "fall of the one-night stand," and the
end of the Swinging Seventies.

Most public health officials had mixed feeling about these developments. On the one hand, the AIDS epidemic was getting public
attention as never before. Our ability to engage in frank and explicit
dialogue with the public, and the acceptance of the important condom message, was becoming much easier. And there was a real
heterosexual threat: if you had sex or shared needles with a partner
who was likely to be infected, you were at real risk. Relatively few
people could be absolutely sure of the history of their current or
past sexual partners. It was important to demythologize the antibody test, to reinforce the messages of risk reduction to self and
others, to persuade more people that knowing whether one was
positive or negative was much better than not knowing. And though
few public health professionals believed that a large-scale breakout
of AIDS would occur in the "general population," we were mostly
all persuaded that there would be slow and persistent seepage of
cases across all ethnic, class, and geographic lines.

Most important of all, the first lessons of the epidemic were those of our vulnerability—that this virus should never be underestimated. Overconfidence was foolish.

And yet the heterosexual panic was a distortion of the actual dangers. It was important to focus on the problem where it really was, but how could that be done without further harming minorities or, as actually began to happen by 1990, losing the attention of the middle class? Might there be a backlash down the road if the middle class decided the epidemic had been, from their perspective, exaggerated? It seemed that our arguments and our messages were being diverted from the groups who most needed them. Otherwise carefully written books, such as Chris Norwood's *Advice for Life: A Woman's Guide to AIDS Risks and Prevention,* did not clearly differentiate among the probabilities based on race, class, and geographic location. The sense of the epidemic that seemed to be gaining acceptance with heterosexuals was that risk was nonselective.

The Health Department's anonymous test sites began to attract more women, but were they the right women? As Ron Sullivan wrote in the *New York Times* in May 1987, "Concern about AIDS in New York City has reached such proportions that increasing numbers of women who are presumably at low risk are seeking to be tested." He noted that at one testing site on the East Side, 40 percent of the people who sought to be tested were women considered at low risk. None tested positive.

Some of my colleagues thought it was not good that we were getting so many "worried well" at test sites. I disagreed. Perhaps many of these people had good reason to worry, even if we labeled them low risk. If they were worried about a fatal infection, wasn't it a legitimate use of public health resources to reassure them? Most important, wasn't the counseling/testing process likely to be the best of all risk-reduction educational processes, and wouldn't more testing beget more testing of higher as well as lower-risk persons? I thought that the answer was yes, and that the appropriate response was to find more creative ways to streamline counseling for lower-risk individuals rather than to discourage them from using the counseling and testing process.

The apogee of the heterosexual panic, from which it then receded, came in early 1988 when William Masters and Virginia Johnson, household names in American sex research, published (with Robert Kolodny) *CRISIS: Heterosexual Behavior in the Age of AIDS.* Alarmist and shrill, the book claimed that "AIDS is now running rampant" in the general heterosexual population, estimated that over three million Americans were infected, and resuscitated old canards about casual contact and transmission.

Had the book appeared just one year earlier, it undoubtedly would have fueled fears about heterosexual transmission. But in 1988, it received only brief and almost universally dismissive attention. It was a mark of how far the media had come in sophistication about the epidemic that journalists, echoing virtually the entire scientific community, destroyed the credibility of the book in a few days. As the *New York Daily News* put it: "Sexperts retreat on AIDS." Ed Edelson wrote: "Sex therapists William Masters and Virginia Johnson waffled yesterday on their controversial claim that AIDS was 'running rampant' in the heterosexual community, admitting it was based more on their beliefs than scientific evidence."

But irresponsible advice came from the opposite direction as well. In January 1988, the influential women's magazine *Cosmopolitan* published an article by psychiatrist Robert E. Gould that dismissed the risk of heterosexual infection and "tells why most women are safe from AIDS." Editor Helen Gurley Brown wrote, "But part of the AIDS mystique, part of the reason we did this article, is that women, who just got their sexual adulthood—all of a sudden were not supposed to have sex any more because it's dangerous. And that just plays into the hands of a whole lot of people who thought that women shouldn't have a sex life anyway. They couldn't be more thrilled that now we're gonna have the daylights scared out of us unnecessarily. But I would say, 'Don't let AIDS ruin your life.'"

Just as the Masters and Johnson hypothesis was damaging in overdrawing the HIV heterosexual threat, the *Cosmopolitan* article was equally damaging in denying the reality of that risk. And both approaches ignored the key point that specific groups of heterosexuals were endangered and needed to know and act upon that knowledge.

The "heterosexual panic" of 1987 changed the milieu of the AIDS epidemic permanently. No longer did the white middle-class public think itself immune or unthreatened. The overreaction and hysteria about greatly exaggerated risks were to pass quite quickly. By 1990, as it became apparent that no middle-class breakout had occurred, the drift began to move again in the other direction: loss of fear, loss of interest in the overall issues of the epidemic.

But the seeds of doubt had been sown, especially in the minds of women. After all, who could be absolutely sure that a former or current partner was completely free of risk? Among men, if anything, the fears of infection by a female sexual partner remained exaggerated out of proportion to what the data supported.

In my view, all these fears, out-of-proportion though they might be, were a constructive development. First, it is important that the risks of infection to heterosexuals be acknowledged. While it now seems clear that there will be no explosion of AIDS throughout the middle-class population, there will be a continued number of heterosexually transmitted cases. The only questions at issue, impossible to answer definitively at this time, are whether this rate of heterosexual cases, outside the high-risk areas and minority groups, will be small or very small, and whether the rate of new cases will increase or has already reached a plateau.

Second, heterosexual fears legitimized frank discussion of AIDS issues, condom use, and related issues among Americans. I used to tell a joke as part of public statements when, as Health Commissioner, I fought for the enactment of strong antismoking legislation in the city: "A woman goes into a drugstore, marches up to the counter and says (loudly) to the clerk, 'Give me a package of condoms and (whispers) a package of cigarettes.'"

Third, the generalized heterosexual concerns undoubtedly made it easier to focus the attention of minority women on their much greater risks, and to engage political and community leadership in coming to grips with the problem.

For men and women, the perceptions of 1987 highlighted a host of other issues that are yet to be resolved.

Was there, or would there yet be, a change in American sexual mores? My own guess is that there has been some moderate change among many heterosexuals regarding the numbers and "casualness" of their sexual partners, and some moderate increase in condom use.

But it is highly unlikely that any major shift in sexual patterns regarding chastity or monogamy or strict adherence to safer sex guidelines has taken place. I think that those changes that did occur in the latter 1980s as a result of AIDS anxiety are not likely to persist through the early 1990s.

And then there are the children of AIDS. In addition to the direct toll of disease and death of infants and children from HIV, many social problems will be created by the deaths of the mothers of uninfected children. New York City alone, by the late 1990s, will have some 10,000–20,000 children whose mothers have died of AIDS—in many, perhaps most, instances these will have been single-parent families. The trauma borne by these children and the concomitant and resultant social problems, not to mention the economic costs of the orphan issue, will be extreme.

The AIDS epidemic has raised many difficult issues of reproductive health for women. An infected woman has about a one-third chance of bearing an infected child (currently, half of those children are dead by 15 months of age; it is expected that most of the others will not survive past early childhood). Those children who are not infected face the prospect of a mother who is now unlikely to survive their childhood. All this is, of course, in a rapidly changing therapeutic context.

Debate continues to rage about the appropriate counsel to be given to HIV-infected women concerning childbearing. The Centers for Disease Control recommends that "pregnancy be deferred." What does this mean in the case of a lifelong infection? Many civil libertarians and women's advocates express concern that HIV-infected women are being pressured to avoid or terminate pregnancy, and this argument takes a volatile racial and ethnic turn because of the overwhelming proportion of black and Hispanic women among those infected.

My own view, as a physician, is that women must be given full and current information about the known risks and consequences and about their own infected or noninfected status. Decisions about pregnancy and abortion should be the woman's own, and she should be supported in those decisions by the medical personnel caring for her. But I would personally find it very difficult to counsel an HIV-infected woman that to conceive or carry to term a fetus was in her own or the future child's best interests.

The reproductive health issues underscore the failure of public health systems to devise a routine system of antibody testing for reproductive-age women, and especially for women early in pregnancy. I believe that with aggressive attention to the issue by doctors and nurses, we could ensure that virtually all women know their antibody status without coercion or mandatory testing. We have not been able to achieve this, because of misguided zeal on the part of those who would protect these women from themselves and thus stand in the path of any attempt to expand testing. This is a travesty of caring for patients.

From the antibody testing of newborns, New York State already has the information showing the infection status of every new mother. To preserve anonymity, it strips the identifiers off all this data, so that even the mother who wants to know the test result cannot. While knowledge of maternal antibody status after a child's birth is not optimal timing, it does have value to a woman with regard to the future welfare of herself and that child and, of course, with regard to future pregnancies. To deny women who want it access to this information (and I believe most would want the test result information which is critical to their health and their children's health), while at the same time making it very difficult for the woman to get a repeat test or to get the information by some other route is, I believe, medical and public health negligence.

The issues of heterosexual transmission of the HIVirus became pivotal to a wide variety of public health and public policy debates. The circumstances of testing of women, infants, and sexual partners is only one set of issues. Even more volatile are the questions of mandatory reporting of infected persons to health departments and the tracing of sexual partners. Though opposition to this has been a political rallying point of homosexual groups, the issues of greatest significance at this point in the epidemic concern heterosexual transmission and the infection of newborns. The partner's "right to know" and the "physician's duty to warn" likewise came into sharper focus as the discussion of heterosexual AIDS developed.

Indeed, the most controversial public policy questions regarding the future conduct of the struggle against AIDS, though they have been most vocally articulated by gay advocacy groups, really reached public consciousness only after the realization, exaggerated though it was, of the threat to heterosexuals.

# 6

## *How Many Infected Among Us?*

When you ask Nature a question, she always gives you an answer. But she may not be giving you the answer to the question that you thought you were asking her.

—Claude Bernard, French scientist/philosopher

A virus does not discriminate. A virus does not know the difference between black and white or straight and gay or male and female. Why doesn't anyone believe that?

—Robert McFarlane, Director of Professional AIDS Education, Memorial Sloan-Kettering Cancer Center, 1990

Answer: Because it's not true.

EPIDEMIOLOGY IS THE STUDY OF DISEASE IN POPULATIONS (RATHER THAN in individuals); it measures and compares trends and changes in disease occurrences and characteristics. By studying a disease's features common to or differing among a sufficiently large number of people, and subjecting the results to statistical analysis, a great deal of information about the disease can be developed rapidly, with confidence in the analytic and predictive power of the information.

But epidemiologic accuracy (Bernard's "answer to the question you thought you were asking") requires understanding in accurate detail both the people affected by the condition and the entire population at risk of the condition. An error in defining or counting either group will produce a faulty analysis.

# Getting the Numbers Right

One of the most difficult problems inherent in understanding the AIDS epidemic is a classical "numerator" problem. During the first five years of the epidemic, we were only able to count cases of AIDS, not the larger numbers of people who were infected with the HIVirus. The long lag time of several years between infection and illness resulted in a perspective on the epidemic that was about five years out of date. Even if all cases of AIDS had been reported completely and quickly to public health authorities, there still remained the problem of those HIV-ill persons whose symptoms did not fulfill the criteria for a formal diagnosis of AIDS. These are usually estimated to be three to four times the number of people diagnosed with AIDS; my personal view is that the actual current ratio of HIV-ill to AIDS may be as high as 5 or even 7 to one, because of medicine's increasing skills in making earlier and more subtle diagnosis of HIV-related illness. Beyond these, of course, are even larger numbers of people infected with the HIVirus, but as yet with no identifiable signs or symptoms of any illness.

In the first five years, the epidemiology of AIDS presented a set of dilemmas. How was one to be sure of capturing a complete and accurate total—all, and only, cases of AIDS, no misdiagnoses? What was the relationship of this total of AIDS cases to another and more important number for predicting the longer-term future of the epidemic, that is, the number and characteristics of all those infected with the HIVirus?

What were the appropriate reference groups by which to describe those who were at risk: homosexuals, intravenous drug users, hemophiliacs, recipients of blood transfusions, heterosexual partners? What about Haitians, exposed health and emergency workers, offspring of infected parents? In some cases there was debate as to whether a group should even be classified as high risk, as a reference against which cases of AIDS should be measured, and then compared to rates among other groups. Should one group, for example, include all Haitians? Only Haitians with a history of drug abuse or homosexual/bisexual behavior? Only Haitians who entered the United States after 1977? Such questions were not only scientifically perplexing; they had important practical applications—for example, to exclude high-risk blood donors in order to protect the blood supply.

And they are fraught with potential and actual political conflict. As late as 1990, when a Food and Drug Administration (FDA) advisory committee recommended excluding all Haitians as donors of blood, there was a major outcry and organized street demonstration condemning this as a racist measure. The FDA was forced to reject the recommendation.

Beyond the difficult problems of deciding whom to include in numerator (affected) and denominator (risk) groups were the equally difficult problems of counting accurately. How many homosexual or bisexual men were there in New York City, or in the country? How many intravenous drug users? How could one estimate the numbers of women who might be sexually at risk?

With the advent of the HIV-antibody test in the spring of 1985 and growing confidence in its accuracy, we theoretically had the tools to develop a current profile of HIV infection without depending on the possibly misleading number of AIDS cases. Even with the important weaknesses in making estimates as described above, it would have been theoretically possible by 1986 or 1987 to begin fighting the battle against AIDS with current topographic maps rather than ancient chart fragments.

This theoretical opportunity, however, never had a ghost of a chance. At a time in the epidemic when we had little or nothing to offer therapeutically to individuals who tested HIV-antibody positive (1985–1987), and with powerful stigmatization concerning AIDS operating in society, broadly based programs of mandatory testing or involuntary screening were strongly opposed.

In New York City, attempts to estimate the size and shape of the early epidemic were hampered by a combination of factors that were perhaps more difficult to deal with than those in any other city. The first factor was the size and diversity of the epidemic, and the populations presumed to be infected. Second was the resistance of the gay community to the widespread use of the antibody test, even voluntarily, and the corresponding hesitancy, at that time, of the New York City and State Health Departments to push more forcefully for greater testing. It was not until August 1989, in fact, that New York's Gay Men's Health Crisis publicly encouraged gay men to voluntarily be tested and to learn their HIV antibody status. The influence of the political definition of the epidemic surpassed the scientific desire to know the full dimensions of infection.

New York City is the only metropolitan area in the United States that is treated as an independent statistical area (independent of the state in which it is located), and which has its own vital statistics system. All New York City Commissioners of Health have felt strongly about the importance of preserving this independent vital statistics system in view of the city's complexity, the importance of its disease patterns and trends, and its fundamental demographic, environmental, and social differences from the rest of the state. To include 13 million upstate residents as part of the denominators of epidemiologic equations seeking to shed light on health issues among 7 million city residents would play havoc with epidemiologic principles. Thus, New York City has jealously guarded its "home rule" in vital statistics.

From the beginning of the epidemic, New York City required and received name reporting of AIDS cases from physicians and hospitals, performed its own surveillance and research, kept its own records, and reported cases and trends to the state and to the CDC only on an anonymous basis. The importance of understanding the epidemic's magnitude, profile, and trends within the city was self-evident.

In the absence of any way to measure the extent of infection until 1985, New York City adopted a system similar to virtually all other jurisdictions, and used reported cases of AIDS as the indicator for tracking the epidemic, not only in the past and present, but also for projecting future trends. By constructing a trend line on the basis of each six-month total of reported cases (all AIDS cases, or all AIDS cases in a particular group), a projection of the number of cases that might be expected some years into the future could be constructed, and then updated semiannually. The overall method for estimating total numbers of AIDS cases, though statistically primitive, proved to be quite accurate, as the epidemic evolved and actually occurring cases could be compared with past projections.

There were important limitations, however, to the benefits of this method. Though it allowed a rather precise definition of one risk group in the epidemic (cases of CDC-defined AIDS), it missed the broader span of HIV illness, an even more important group for purposes of planning future needed services and estimating the burdens that would fall upon health and social service agencies.

Counting cases of full-blown AIDS also did not help us understand the natural history of the progression of HIV illness (the proportion of infected individuals who would become ill, and at what rate). Most important from a public health perspective, because it was five to ten years out of date and represented an unknown proportion of those infected, the number of AIDS cases was a very poor proxy for the actual progress of the epidemic of infection. Recent movement of the virus by neighborhood, gender, race, ethnicity, social class, or behavior patterns could not be measured directly.

Thus, though the department based its measurements of the epidemic on reported cases of AIDS, there was a strong need to estimate the currently unmeasurable number of New Yorkers who were apparently healthy but actually infected with the virus, and who would become the HIV-ill and AIDS cases of future years.

The problem was most acute with regard to homosexual and bisexual men. No one had any reliable idea of the number of such men in New York City, even if one could arrive at a definition that would have a relationship to relative risk of infection. Further, no one, including gay organizations, could design a study to measure the size of this population reliably.

It was decided to use Alfred Kinsey's 1948 conclusion that 10 percent of American men are more or less exclusively homosexual. The accuracy of the Kinsey data was much challenged, it was forty years old, and it had never been validated by other studies. However, no other data was available. Thus this highly speculative percentage was applied to the entire male adult population of New York City, and a resultant estimate of up to 500,000 men who have sex with men (the formal label of CDC's category) was arrived at. Note that the Kinsey figure itself would not include most bisexual men, about whom virtually no data exists.

The proportion of gay men who were actually infected with the HIVirus in 1985 was also very difficult to estimate. Several small sample surveys of gay men from New York and San Francisco suggested that up to 60 percent were infected with the virus. But there was no assurance that the men in those sample surveys were truly representative of the entire homosexual/bisexual male population of New York, and there was good reason to speculate that the men in those early surveys might well represent a much higher risk group than did the gay population at large. Indeed, succeeding surveys have shown that the prevalence of HIV infection in gay men in New York is much more like 25–35 percent rather than 60 percent.

The methods of deriving both the "up to 500,000" and the 60 percent components of the initial estimate contained the weakness that they made no allowance for differential levels of risk in varying subgroups of homosexuals, even beyond the great probability that both components were significantly overestimated. But with those inherent limitations, the estimate was derived of somewhere between 150,000 and 300,000 infected homosexual and bisexual men in New York City in 1985; and 200,000 or 250,000 was the rough figure generally employed.

With intravenous drug users, there was more data, but it was also far from ironclad. Various estimates from health and law enforcement sources placed the numbers of heroin injectors in New York City at about 200,000, though again that overall figure does not distinguish among widely varying degrees of risk behavior. Recent studies of rates of HIV infection among intravenous drug users estimated a prevalence of infection from 50 to 60 percent. In contrast to the initial estimate of 60 percent infection among gay men, the range of 50–60 percent prevalence of HIV infection among intravenous drug users has been repeatedly validated in various studies since 1985. To construct the initial estimate of HIV infection among intravenous drug users, the high-end figures of 250,000 intravenous drug users, among whom 60 percent were infected, was employed.

Thus, with major components of about 250,000 infected men who have sex with men, roughly 150,000 infected intravenous drug users, and up to 50,000 non-drug-using heterosexuals estimated to be infected, a total estimate was arrived at of around 400,000.

This estimate was derived and published shortly before I became Commissioner of Health in May 1986. It immediately gained great currency in the media (400,000 persons is an impressive number), without of course careful explanation by the media of all the fine print necessary to understand the many caveats as to its accuracy. No one voiced serious public doubts as to the accuracy of the numbers, there were no competing estimates offered, and it clearly fit the agendas of all groups (including those in public health) attempting to draw public attention to the seriousness and magnitude of the epidemic.

Within a few months the United States Public Health Service had issued an estimate of 1–1.5 million infected people in the nation. Because New York City accounted for about one-third of the country's AIDS cases, the infection estimates seemed to dovetail. From that point onward, not only was there little public skepticism about the initial New York City estimates, but increasingly there were a series of vested interests engaged in defending and promoting them.

## The Consequences of the Estimates

I probably did as much as anyone, perhaps more, to lock in the "400,000 infected New Yorkers" number. I came to my post as commissioner determined to put the department in a much more active posture in the AIDS epidemic, expand prevention, counseling, and testing services as rapidly as possible, and, perhaps most of all, raise the level of awareness and involvement of New Yorkers about the seriousness of the epidemic for all facets of the city's life.

I used the platform that comes with the office of the Health Commissioner to speak out as often and as visibly as I could. My strategy was that to the extent I could convince the public of the horrors projected in a realistic appraisal of the epidemic, the easier it would be to increase resources for AIDS prevention and AIDS services from City Hall, Albany, and Washington.

It is my strong conviction that an essential component of effective public health communication is a determination to present the best, most current, and unvarnished information that science can provide. This requires a willingness to alter, without embarrassment, prior predictions or explanations as new data invalidate earlier statements or positions. Rather than eroding public confidence, it seems to me that this is the way to gain credibility and public confidence. This is particularly important in public health, where, on most occasions, the news you bring is neither pleasant nor welcome.

While the 400,000 estimate was the best (and only) estimate we had, it had disquieting weaknesses from the start. Some had to do with the shaky nature of the basic figures upon which the estimates were constructed. But there were other ways in which the estimate "did not compute."

As we began to learn more about HIV infection's progression to AIDS—and the rate of that progression—the infection estimates appeared widely discordant with the numbers of AIDS cases. The numbers of expected versus observed cases of AIDS just did not match. For example, if there were 400,000 infected New Yorkers in 1987, and even if only 100,000 of them had been infected as early as 1982, then we should have expected some 20,000 cumulative cases of AIDS (from research that showed that 15–25 percent of infected persons developed full-blown AIDS within five years of infection). But we actually had received fewer than 8,300 reported adult cases through 1987. The department carried out validation studies showing there was no large proportion of unreported cases. Where were the "missing" cases? It was likely that the estimate itself was grossly overstated.

The department's staff was increasingly uncomfortable with the publicity that the 400,000 figure was getting. Both they and I were in ambivalent positions: they had derived the figures; I was making them as visible as I could; and though the estimates were the best we had, none of us was completely confident of their accuracy.

By the spring of 1987, I had asked department staff to do two things to improve the situation: to reopen a series of validation studies (to make sure we were not "missing" a large proportion of cases; these reviews showed no great falloff in reporting efficiency), and to try to develop an improved method of estimating the number of those who were infected with the virus.

Within a year, the department had developed a new and better estimation method, one whose strength lay in completely avoiding the necessity of estimating the size of the population of homosexual and bisexual men. The method was based on a comparison of cases of AIDS in New York City and San Francisco, and upon a much more confident estimate of the number of gay and bisexual men in San Francisco arrived at by their Department of Health. The accuracy of such a comparison, of course, depended on the epidemics in New York and San Francisco being similar in their relevant aspects. Despite some uncertainties, the new methodology allowed a base for estimating the number of infected New Yorkers that was much more likely to be accurate than the former estimate, and the resulting estimate gave a better fit to several other sets of data.

The new study cut the previously estimated 400,000 infected New Yorkers in half. The public announcement cutting in half the estimate of infected New Yorkers caused an immediate, intense, and protracted response of protest from New York's gay community.

# Politics and the Numbers

By 1988, all groups concerned had begun to argue for a more cohesive approach in New York City to planning for the epidemic and marshaling the wide range of resources needed to meet it. The Department of Health had made three attempts at describing the future of the epidemic, but only within the context of city government, and without the level of detail and sophistication that was clearly needed.

Thus, in March 1988, a broadly based group, the New York City AIDS Task Force, came together under the umbrella of the local voluntary Health Systems Agency. With myself as chairman, funding both from the city and voluntary agencies, a paid executive director and staff, and membership drawn from the entire spectrum of public, private, and voluntary organizations dealing with AIDS, the task force was formed to produce a plan that could reach beyond the governmental response. Its primary purpose was to define the needed resources for dealing with the epidemic, and then to advocate for their commitment.

The first work group of the Task Force to get busy was charged with laying out the epidemiologic parameters, the current and projected pattern of AIDS cases, and the profiles of infection on which all other projections of service needs would be based. The group depended heavily on the Department of Health for basic data and staff support, but was entirely independent in reaching its conclusions. Its work estimating the numbers of HIV-infected New Yorkers ran parallel to the department's own internal efforts—both came up with similar estimates of infected New Yorkers, an estimate almost half as small as the previously estimated 400,000.

When I saw the group's draft report, I realized that it would include the revised estimate of infected New Yorkers—a number that had not yet been publicly released. My initial thought was that making the first announcement of the reduced estimate of the number of HIV-infected persons in New York City at the AIDS Task Force meeting would cause immense public confusion that would be difficult to unscramble. The question to me would be: Why is the "official" Department of Health estimate still 400,000 when the Task Force has revised it downward by a factor of two?

I saw no better choice than to organize a press conference for early the following week at the Health Department, at which we would release the new estimates and discuss their implications. I assumed, naïvely as it turned out, that while there would be some skepticism about the numbers, the downward revision would generally be taken as good news.

I informed the Mayor, through First Deputy Mayor Brezenoff, my routine reporting channel, and set my public affairs staff to work alerting the media and preparing for the conference. At this point I made what was to prove a serious mistake. I neglected to call key AIDS advocates to tell them what I would be saying at the press conference. The Deputy Director of Gay Men's Health Crisis had already seen a draft of the Task Force's report, describing the reduced estimates, and I assumed incorrectly that had there been major concerns from that quarter I would have heard them.

I also leaned too heavily on my own conviction that "epidemiology was not negotiable." Convinced that we had objectively arrived at a much more accurate estimate than the previous one, I blinded myself to the possibility that others would see the issue primarily in political, rather than scientific, terms. I was to pay dearly for that oversight. While prior discussion of the revisions we were about to announce would not have satisfied those who did not want to believe the figures, and while I would never have agreed to withhold information that was important for the public to have, prior consultation would have avoided the resentment among those who were blindsided by the announcement and would have reduced the appeal of conspiratorial theories regarding the motives and methods of arriving at the reduced estimates.

The Health Department board room was packed with print and

electronic journalists. The gist of our announcement had leaked out to the press, and the *New York Times* had carried a story that morning with the headline, "New York City Cuts Its Estimate in Half for AIDS Infection."

I stressed that the new estimates would in no way lower the investment or action required over the next few years to cope with the epidemic, pointed out that we were not reducing our projections of the 43,000 cases of AIDS to be expected by the end of 1991, and that the estimates made no assumptions about the number of gay or bisexual men living in New York City.

Gay advocates bitterly attacked the new estimates. Their arguments were that the Health Department (more specifically, I) had failed to consult with them either out of disrespect for their views or to deliberately catch them unawares. It was alleged that the lowered estimates were intended to downplay the epidemic's importance so that the Koch administration could reduce its budgetary expenditures. The advocates charged that the estimates were changed as part of a political plot to diminish the power of the gay community itself.

The first charge was inaccurate in spirit, but not defensible in substance. In my first two years as Health Commissioner, I had enjoyed a productive relationship with the gay advocacy organizations. My contacts began before I was sworn in, when a gay friend held a private dinner at which I met about twenty community leaders. Despite claims by the gay community that the Koch Administration was not putting enough effort or money into the epidemic, I had been able to work collaboratively with them on many issues and, I believe, was initially generally viewed favorably by most gay leaders as well as the rank-and-file.

The battle over the revised estimates changed all that. Feelings of betrayal on their part and anger on my part over the disingenuous nature of allegations that I had falsified science for political ends, soured all but a few of the professional relationships and personal friendships between myself and leaders of gay advocacy groups. The nascent activist group ACT-UP found a figure against which to coalesce its anger and build its organization.

The second charge, that I was fudging data to serve some political purpose, was particularly repugnant. We had developed the data objectively, and I had reviewed it with my strongest-held conviction as a physician: to face the realities of the data, no matter what its implications for yourself or others. Ed Koch had nothing to do with the development of the estimates; I had communicated them to him only after we were satisfied that they were the best that could be achieved, and he had never, on any issue, asked me to slant any of my public health recommendations to make his political life more comfortable.

I also knew that, in the political environment of New York City, the charges leveled against the infection estimates would be widely believed in the gay community. Their credence was further enhanced by one of those bizarre coincidences that seem to fulfill Murphy's Law.

State Comptroller Edward V. Regan had been working on a report blasting New York City as underresponding to the epidemic. I had seen a draft of his report several weeks earlier. Its science was poor, its tone alarmist, and its conclusions and finger pointing were simplistic. (However, his argument had an important kernel of truth. All of us, everywhere in the city, the state, and the country, had been less than prepared and had underresponded.) Totally by coincidence, Mr. Regan issued his report on the same day as my press conference announcing the lowered infection estimates. I first realized his report had been issued when a reporter asked me at the press conference whether my estimates were not just a gambit to offset the Regan report. I knew that, for those who wanted to see it that way, there was no possibility of belief that the two processes were entirely unconnected, which they were.

A variety of indices gave us confidence that it was relevant to compare the gay/bisexual populations of New York and San Francisco for purposes of determining risk: the epidemic began at roughly the same time in the two cities, the rate of appearance of new cases among gay and bisexual men was similar, the decrease in transmission of HIV among gay men as the decade proceeded (signaled by a marked decline in the occurrence of other sexually transmitted diseases) was parallel, and the methods of surveillance protocols for risk classification were comparable, with a history of close and ongoing contact between the epidemiologists in both Health Departments.

The greatest weakness in the comparability argument was the difference in the racial and ethnic composition of gay/bisexual populations in the two cities, with New York having a much larger proportion of black and Hispanic gay/bisexual men compared to San Francisco. There was no data to bear on how this might influence infection risk, if at all, however, and in our view it was clearly a much smaller flaw in the new methodology than the Kinsey hypothesis or the unknown size of the gay/bisexual population had been in the old.

In all the clamor, what was lost sight of was that any of these estimates were just that—estimates—and that all had to be treated skeptically, and continually examined against new or corollary data for revision when necessary. For a time I could not understand why such intense hostility accompanied a set of numbers that were admittedly imprecise, that were explicitly not the yardsticks of planning for services, and that ought to have been seen as one of the very few pieces of good news in the AIDS environment of 1988. I was convinced that we had come up with a much more accurate picture of the extent of infection, and that other observers would soon move in our direction of lowering initial estimates of the infected population. (As indeed they did; we received almost no argument from epidemiologists or public health experts around the country concerning our revised figures.) In that conviction I missed the forest for the trees.

What the fierce opposition was really about was the third line of argument—that the lowered estimates were a plot to diminish the size and importance of the gay community itself. The opposition was a matter of sexual politics. No matter how I stressed that the new methodology avoided relying on an estimate of the number of gay/bisexual men in New York City, the gay advocates could not view the 200,000 figure in any other way.

While I had written off any hope of working productively with ACT-UP itself, I wanted to rebuild relationships with the more constructive advocacy organizations, feeling that we shared a more common agenda. Within several months, time began to heal the breach caused by the reduced estimate, especially as it became evident that our new estimate was indeed more accurate. I had several meetings with these organizations, and accepted an invitation to speak before an open forum at the Lesbian and Gay Community Center in late November 1988. The *Gay Community News* reported the festivities accurately:

Joseph began the evening by outlining to a tense and nearly completely hostile audience the future trends in the epidemic, which he said was moving away from white, gay men in Manhattan and towards IV-drug users and their sex partners, most of whom are Black and Latino, and who live in poor neighborhoods in Brooklyn, Queens, and the Bronx. The meeting's question and answer period quickly degenerated into an exchange of insults and accusations, with ACT UP members calling Joseph insensitive, deceitful and murderous, and Joseph countering with charges of harassment, threats, lies and stupidity on the part of ACT UP. Joseph dismissed the suggestion that he resign, but repeatedly invited audience members to lobby Mayor Koch for his dismissal.

"You're a liar and a fraud and a self-promoting demagogue, and the meeting is over," Joseph said calmly before walking out of the Center flanked by his two bodyguards nearly two and a half hours after the ordeal had begun. He was responding to an accusation that his department's acceptance of $500,000 from the Centers for Disease Control to investigate the validity of its own epidemiology is tantamount to corruption. The questioner, Ortez Alderson, who has represented ACT UP previously at a meeting with Joseph, began his question by comparing Stephen Joseph to Nazi torturer Joseph Mengele. Dr. Joseph denied the accusation of corruption and denounced the comparison. There are currently no plans for another forum.

Though the breach with gay community leadership was painful, I was confident that a short period of time would lead to the more general realization that the new estimates were accurate, and would discredit the various conspiratorial theories surrounding them. This indeed proved to be so, with regard to the public health community and the general population. Regarding ACT-UP, however, I could not have been more wrong.

As I stood gazing at an AIDS education poster produced by the State Department of Health in 1987, I asked my staff what its slogan: "AIDS Does Not Discriminate," meant. The poster showed a group of people intended to represent a wide spectrum of ethnicity, age group, class, and sexual preference—a white man in a hard hat, a black man with a stethoscope, a schoolteacherish looking woman, an Asian child, a pretty young Caucasian girl. Was the state suggesting that the physician was a closeted homosexual? Or that the school teacher was an IV drug user? Or that the child had received a contaminated blood transfusion? No. The state was suggesting that every American was equally vulnerable to AIDS.

In fact, precisely the opposite is true. The HIVirus is an exquisitely discriminating virus. The slogan that AIDS does not discriminate is exactly wrong. The HIVirus discriminates in precisely who it is going to attack and where it is going to go.

The virus's discrimination was at the heart of its political controversy: very few people involved with AIDS were willing to admit to themselves or others that the HIVirus had preferentially attacked some groups—male homosexuals, IV drug users, and the partners of both—and left others much less affected. Heterosexual middle-class Americans living outside large cities who did not use drugs, and whose sexual partners were not drug injectors or bisexual men, were unlikely to encounter the disease except through highly improbable bad luck—a contaminated transfusion in the early days of the epidemic. Yet both official and advocacy public education campaigns seemed intent on showing that anyone at any time could become infected, without taking account of the wildly differing probabilities of exposure to infection depending upon who you were, where you lived, what you did, and who you did it with.

In particular, AIDS activists found any reference to the virus's ability to discriminate as a not very veiled justification of discrimination against those who were infected. More than any other characteristic, the virus's discrimination hampered our ability to attack its spread effectively.

# ACT-UP in Action

I had first come across the AIDS Coalition To Unleash Power at a
CDC-sponsored conference in Atlanta during February 1987. There
I observed men wearing the ACT-UP symbol, a pink triangle (the
badge that the Nazis had forced homosexuals to wear, but now with
the triangle inverted, point up), shouting their dissent from the audience when any comment by one of the scientific presenters dis-
pleased them. Costumed as concentration camp inmates, a small
group circulated through the meeting rooms and hallways, drama-
tizing their contention that Federal and scientific lack of progress on
AIDS was genocidal. Their slogan was "Silence=Death," and they
were clearly resolved not to remain silent.

I had heard of their formation and of some of their early street
demonstrations in New York over the past months. My reaction was
a mixture of empathy for their activism and their courage, skepticism at the free-floating anger and vagueness of their demands
(which, in those early days, were generally a blanket condemnation
of all existing AIDS efforts as inadequate coupled with demands
that "more be done"), and concern regarding the unknown future
directions in which their rage and energy would spill.

One of their leading founders, the playwright Larry Kramer, was
well known for his unremitting hostility to the Mayor and to the
city's efforts regarding AIDS, and also well known for his creativity
with words and protest. I encountered Mr. Kramer for the first time
when I was giving a talk on AIDS at Riverside Church in Manhattan. As I began to speak, a figure paraded down the center aisle
holding aloft a sign saying "Lies." I ignored the distraction, and
continued on. Mr. Kramer became progressively angrier, and began
shouting "He's lying," and, during the discussion period, exhorted

the audience to "not listen to this Killer Wimp." I didn't know it then, but this first encounter was to be the model for my public confrontations with ACT-UP months later: me trying to keep going through my prepared presentation or response to questions, they trying to shout me down.

In the first half of 1988, ACT-UP had increasingly focused its street demonstrations and leafleting against the city administration. The estimates controversy gave them a focus against which to co-alesce, and I was it.

It began largely along rhetorical lines. Posters and stickers were pasted on lampposts and mailboxes around the city, proclaiming that "The AIDS Estimates Are A Lethal Lie," and "Stephen Joseph Has Blood on His Hands" (superimposed on a crimson hand print; in another version the bloody hand was identified as Ed Koch's). A chanting demonstration in front of the Health Department labeled me a murderer and urged that I resign.

The next action was a sit-in at the Health Department. I was away from the building when twelve ACT-UP protesters burst into the executive offices, occupying the office of a Deputy Commissioner and demanding a meeting with me. I sent word that I would never meet under that sort of duress, and urged them to leave peacefully and schedule a meeting under mutually agreeable conditions. Events then followed a predictable path: they refused to leave, I had the police arrest them for criminal trespass, the arrests were carried out ritualistically, they were booked and released.

Less than a week later, they were back. This time the confrontation was much uglier.

I was chairing a meeting in my office of a number of persons from around the city who were helping us create what would eventually emerge as an important public-private partnership: the $11 million Aaron Diamond Research Laboratory for basic research on the AIDS virus. Suddenly, through a side door, burst eleven ACT-UP members, complete with video camera and lawyer, screaming demands, obscenities, and incomprehensible questions. They surrounded the conference table and shouted that they were not leaving until I met with them and satisfied their demands.

I adjourned the meeting, apologized to my colleagues for the interruption, and told the ACT-UP demonstrators that they already knew that I did not respond to hysterical demands or intimidation, and that I was leaving the office to allow them to cool down and leave quietly, or face a replay of the arrests of the preceding week. The screaming demonstrators blocked my path to the door, and there was some mild pushing and shoving as I tried to leave and they tried to keep me in. I reached the door, went into an adjoining office, composed myself, consulted with key staff, called the Mayor's office to inform him, and once again called the police to arrest the trespassers. I then went back into my office and sat down at my conference table, where the demonstrators had installed themselves. My thought was that I might thus avert any potential physical damage to the contents of the office, and that by sitting there but remaining absolutely silent and not responding to their shouts, I might keep the situation relatively calm until the police arrived (Department of Health security personnel were already in the area).

My silence in the face of their screaming and invective seemed to infuriate them further, especially one mustached and sunglassed young man wearing a red dress and high heels, who later sent me an inscribed photograph of the two of us sitting at the end of my conference table. The inscription said: "Stevie Dearest—Thanks for hanging out with us this day; it was just too much fun!!! Let's do it again real soon, huh?!? Ever, Spree."

The police arrived, the demonstrators refused to leave, they were arrested "peacefully," and were again booked and released.

This time I decided to press charges, and the Manhattan District Attorney indicted the eleven for criminal trespass. When the case came to trial nine months later, the demonstrators entered a plea of not guilty by reason of necessity: that the only way open to them to counter my actions in changing the estimates of HIV infection in the city, and my failure in my public health duty in the AIDS epidemic, was for them to take illegal action. The eleven called me as a witness for the defense (!), and kept me on the stand for the better part of two days, attempting to make a show trial and turn the proceedings into a referendum on my actions rather than their own.

In her written opinion finding all the defendants guilty of third degree criminal trespass, Judge Laura Drager concluded that "this court does not doubt that the defendants entered Dr. Joseph's office with a moral conviction that their action was necessary and justified. But moral conviction is not a defense to criminal action. It is commonly conceded that the exercise of a moral judgment based upon individual standards does not carry with it legal justification or immunity from punishment for breach of the law. Civil disobedience has a well-recognized place in the history of our country and the world, but those who engage in such actions must understand that unless the law they violate is unconstitutional they will bear the consequences of their actions."

The defendants were sentenced to several days of city sanitation duty. I do not know whether the sentences were ever served.

Several days after the second sit-in, I sent a letter to ACT-UP saying that I would meet with three of their representatives under the following conditions: a one-hour meeting, at the end of which they would leave voluntarily, with no demonstrations in the vicinity of the Health Department on the day of the meeting. There was some back and forth (they wanted a video camera and press at the meeting; I said no camera and no reporters but that I would allow tape recording of the meeting). The meeting was held in early September, but it was not productive.

ACT-UP's tactics of harassment in August and September 1988 shifted to two major channels: my public appearances and my personal life.

From this point forward, at most public appearances that I made (presentations, lectures, panels, etc.) ACT-UP members were in the audience. Their tactics consisted of first trying to shout me down when I tried to speak, and then shouting charges and hostile questions during the discussion period. My own tactic was to keep going and not let them interrupt me. Because I usually had a microphone it was not possible for them to drown me out. This seemed to frustrate and infuriate them. Because of the threats of personal violence I was generally accompanied to public functions by two police detectives. I felt somewhat embarrassed by this, and it became something of a game between my secretary and me to try and decide if "tonight I should have police protection or not." On only one occasion were the hecklers able to stop me from speaking: at a small evening seminar at Queens College the protesters actually outnumbered the rest of the audience, and I just never got off the ground. On all the other occasions, I made it through and said what I had come to say.

Some incidents were not as benign. At a lecture at the New York Public Library, the discussion degenerated into screaming and shouted insults from the protesters. When a middle-aged woman stood up and angrily confronted one of the protesters, he punched her in the face.

On another occasion, ACT-UP members were waiting on the street for me as I tried to enter the Ford Foundation building for a meeting. As they followed and surrounded me, one of them squeezed into the revolving door compartment with me. Security personnel prevented them from storming the lobby and elevator.

This public harassment, which was to wax and wane over the next two years, left me angry but determined not to lose my temper or to shout back. It was important to me that public health policy not be held hostage to street theater, nor that the shrillness of protest determine my own actions. I do not believe that any continued or expanded protest by ACT-UP would have ever led me to resign.

Beginning shortly after the release of the infection estimates, and lasting for several months, there was also a much more disturbing personal aspect to the harassment. This consisted of obscene and threatening phone calls and mail.

The phone calls began first, and were obviously orchestrated. The pattern was for most calls to start about midnight and continue at intervals of every minute or so for an hour or more, and then to resume after a lapse of several hours.

Most calls featured an anonymous voice (several of which I came to recognize) whispering or shouting, "murderer" or "resign" or some variation on that theme. Others were more sinister, promising some unspecified danger. A large number were obscene, with either the heavy breathing/moaning variant or some more explicit scenario. The worst of these were several addressed to my wife. A number were overtly threatening: "We're going to get you," or "We'll crush you if you don't resign," or "We know where you are and we'll get you." All were anonymous.

This went on, intermittently, for some weeks. I was unwilling to leave the phone off the hook, since I sometimes got middle-of-the-night calls about some health situation in the city, and prided myself on my availability at all times in cases of emergency. The police put a tap and trace on the phone, and we recorded some of the calls. They identified one telephone belonging to a student at Columbia University as the source of a number of the calls. The calls tapered off and eventually ceased.

Much of the hate mail was sent in mid-October, with ACT-UP logo stickers from Washington, D.C., where ACT-UP was holding a demonstration against the Food and Drug Administration. Some of the messages were clear indications of a deep and sick rage:

"The revised AIDS statistics are lie (sic). Soon we'll be in Washington, D.C. but we'll be back . . . and we won't leave you alone until you crack."

"Resign, resign. Does it thrill you to know how many people hate you and would trip you in the street if they had the chance?"

Addressed to: Steven the Pig Joseph, Commie of Health: "I fuck yo wife! No you idiot this is not the Steven Joseph Memorial (mailed from Washington on a Lincoln Memorial postcard) but you could always drop dead."

In a profile article, the *New York Times* had printed my wife's name. From this, the protesters were able to get my home address and our phone number, which had been listed under her name. One evening in September, I walked down my street to find my brownstone apartment building ringed with police and demonstrators, who were screaming and waving the usual signs. This occasion was the closest I came to losing control of my emotions. I confronted one demonstrator, pushed up against him, and spewed a string of obscenities. If the police had not been there to pull me off, I believe I would have hit him, and thus lost all that I had been working to retain. The next morning, when I left my building, I found slogans painted and posters cemented over the entry door and front steps.

These personal attacks and threats and the assault on my home evoked far more anger in me than did the more public protests. It was also difficult to know how seriously to take the threats, veiled or direct. I expect others have had the same experience: you begin by denying the possible risk of real danger or harm, move on to worrying seriously that indeed someone might be deranged enough to actually attack you or your family, think of the ways that you can protect yourself and them, and then finally realize that both the unpredictable act and the planned assault are very difficult to avert, so you go on about your business.

In the end, what was most disturbing about the ACT-UP campaign was its demonstration of how easily radical dissent can slide into fascism when its own tolerance for dissent disappears. Their brownshirt tactics increasingly confused their own perspective with the only "allowable" perspective; any other point of view was to be shouted down as not only "wrong" but "evil." This, in my view, is a tragic inversion of what the AIDS activists and advocates had initially set out to do: fight bigotry and closed-mindedness.

What of the estimates themselves?

Less than a week after the controversy erupted, on July 26, 1988, the Mayor sent me a memo saying he would like to bring together a few top consultants from around the country to review the estimates. We were able to pull together an excellent committee, consisting of the best professionals from around the nation in relevant fields.

The group's report, submitted in February 1989, concluded that the Department's methodology for estimating the number of HIV-infected New Yorkers was solidly grounded and reasonable.

I made no attempt to conceal my delight that the expert panel had found that the estimates which had drawn such fire were, as I said to the *New York Times,* "right on the money." By the time the report was issued, of course, much of the more sensationalistic popular and media debate was well past, and apart from an occasional aberration (such as a garbled article by Kristin Loomis in the *Village Voice* in April 1989 entitled, "Voodoo Statistics: the Health Department's AIDS Mess"), the furor was behind us. Over succeeding months the infection estimates from most of the country began to slide downward, and the U.S. Public Health Service estimate, which had been put at 1–1.5 million nationwide in 1986, was quietly rephrased as 1 million in 1989, then 750,000 to 1 million in 1990.

So what was it all about? One is left disturbed that a legitimate scientific effort would be so suspected of political manipulation; one is sobered at the difficulty of communicating ranges of uncertainty and margins of error. But it would be naïve to expect the responses to have been much different with regard to an issue with the emotional and magical power of AIDS. And once again, the controversy demonstrated that it was the political and social definitions, and not the scientific or medical ones, that drove policy debate in the epidemic.

The estimates controversy did set in motion a bitter struggle between myself and ACT-UP. They saw me as an arch-devil deliberately insensitive to the needs of people with AIDS, perhaps all gay people; I saw them as a group of bigots unable to tolerate any views but their own, and unable to place their own interests in any relative context of competing needs. It was a struggle that was to flare again a year later, over a much more substantive issue, the public health approach to the epidemic.

Almost obscured in the decibels of the controversy over the infection estimates was the point that we had tried to make at the outset and on which the AIDS advocates, including ACT-UP, and I held common ground: that the most urgent need now was for expanded resources and services; infection estimates had little light to shed on those difficult questions.

Perhaps Bruce Vladeck, president of the United Hospital Fund in New York, had said it best:

> Realistically, however, there is no way that New York City's health care system, as now configured, can provide such comprehensive care for "even" 200,000 persons. It is already reeling from the burden of caring for 7,000 active AIDS cases. Furthermore, there is no way, with current resources, that it could possibly identify all 200,000 persons; the capacity for testing and counseling, while expanding rapidly, is still inadequate. Finally, at current prices, the cost of administering AZT to only one-quarter of the 200,000—roughly $400 million a year, not including physician and laboratory costs or the costs of treating the complications the drug often induces—is prohibitive.

From the viewpoint of those planning and developing health services, whether the river is 200 feet deep or 400 feet deep, it is well past flood stage, and even if we could all agree on what kinds of levees to construct, no one would have any idea of where to get all the sandbags.

# 7

## *Storm Over Montreal*

ONE JOURNALIST DESCRIBED IT THIS WAY:

When New York City Health Commissioner Stephen Joseph was introduced to the hall of 1,000 people at the Fifth International Conference on AIDS in Montreal in early June, about 25 members of the gay activist group ACT-UP stood and turned their backs to him. They unfastened their watches and held them in the air, a powerful symbol that time was passing and that people were dying.

"KOCH'S HIT MAN!"

Joseph stepped up to the podium. As almost everyone in attendance already knew, he was going to use this opportunity to introduce a proposal to begin mandatory reporting and contact tracing of HIV-positive people. "New York City recently recorded its 20,000th case of . . ."

"IT'S A LIE!"

"COMMISSIONER OF DEATH!"

"200 NEEDLES FOR 500,000 ADDICTS!"

The volume on Joseph's microphone seemed to increase just slightly. He kept reading.

"DO SOMETHING!"

"ASSHOLE!"

"SHAME! SHAME! SHAME!"

At that moment Joseph broke from the text of his speech and said to the crowd, "I hope you'll excuse me. It seems I've brought my cheering section with me from New York City."

—Jeffrey Goodell, *Seven Days*, July 12, 1989

Thus went my address to the Fifth Annual Conference on AIDS, held in Montreal in June 1989, one of a series of meetings held in New York, Paris, Washington, and Stockholm. As part of the crash approach to understanding the public health problems of the epidemic, a large, diverse, and somewhat fragmented meeting had begun to be held annually at which new information from all over the world could be analyzed and exchanged, leap-frogging the usual process of communication through published scientific journals. If the conference series paid a price in lessened scientific polishing of data presented before publication, it gained a value in rapid and extensive interchange of new developments. The meetings were exhaustively covered by the world press and, beginning with the 1987 Washington Conference, AIDS advocacy groups had begun to play an important part in the discussions and policy debates.

With some 9,000 expected attendees, the Montreal Conference was to take place against a background of dramatic new advances in AIDS treatment, and a rising tide of radical activism by advocates dissatisfied with the pace and quality of action by medical researchers, the pharmaceutical industry, and government.

When Ivan Head, the Canadian organizer of the conference, asked me to make one of the plenary presentations on the first full day of the meeting, I thought this would afford an ideal opportunity to urge an enhanced public health response to the epidemic. Here was a globally visible scientific forum where, I reasoned, the fullest discussion of policy options should be encouraged in open debate, and where new or provocative ideas would have the broadest possible exposure.

I felt obliged to warn Ivan that any presentation I would make would probably be accompanied by some heckling and protest. For the last year or more, ACT-UP had been demonstrating at every public occasion on which I spoke in New York, and I was sure that they would see the opportunity in Montreal in much the same light as I did: to advance their own agenda. Ivan said not to give it a thought, that they understood that there would be a series of protest demonstrations at the conference, but that the organizers and the Canadian government were prepared to contain them.

My wife and I flew to Montreal on Saturday afternoon, June 3, to enjoy the city before the ceremonial opening session on Sunday afternoon, to confer with colleagues, and to take the temperature of the conference, including the tenor of the protest activities.

I would have to return to New York early Tuesday morning after my Monday morning presentation (it was budget negotiation time in New York). I knew that my new proposals would receive heavy television coverage on Monday, and because I wanted a more comprehensive reporting in New York than sound bites on television, I gave an advance copy of my prepared remarks to several city newspaper reporters who would not be traveling to Montreal, with their agreement that they would not use the material until Monday, its date of delivery. I hoped that this would also serve to increase the interest in what I had to say. In this I was not disappointed, at least insofar as ACT-UP was concerned.

The conference registration sessions gave indications of the confrontations to come, with massive police security facing off groups of demonstrators, and with rumors about false registration passes, packing of the vast conference center by demonstrators, and plans for disruption of the opening ceremonies.

In fact, the opening ceremonies were delayed by more than two hours, as gay activists entered the hall, occupied the stage, and refused to budge until given assurance that attendance at the session would be unrestricted and open to all, whether registered at the conference or not.

Those of us who were scheduled to be plenary speakers were protectively grouped in a waiting area, prior to taking our places, while Ivan Head, security officials, the Canadian Minister of Health, and the security details of Prime Minister Brian Mulroney and President Kenneth Kuanda of Zambia (both of whom were to address the session) huddled and haggled with each other and with the activists concerning demands and security risks. For a while it looked as if Prime Minister Mulroney would cancel his appearance; the Ministry of Health people were greatly embarrassed at what looked like an inability of the Canadian government to control the situation and the crowd.

The conference organizers then made a series of unfortunate concessions that gave the demonstrators control of the front seating sections, where they would be best placed to heckle speakers while in television focus. The Mounties and other security personnel were understandably upset. Eventually ceremonies began, with the featured participants clustered off to one side of the stage and surrounded by security personnel.

The demonstrators' theater was colorful and deafening. Waving banners and signs, shouting slogans, and heckling all the speakers (beginning with denunciations of the Prime Minister for "doing nothing," and carrying through to President Kuanda, who gave a moving address and plea for compassion, describing the death of his son from AIDS, but who made the AIDSpeak error of referring to "victims of AIDS," for which he was hissed).

By any standards, the opening session was a shambles.

As the New York ACT-UP contingent was very visible during the demonstration and in the streets surrounding the conference, I knew that I would have a challenge on the following morning, and resolved to follow my New York practice of not letting any noise level stop me from delivering my remarks.

On Monday morning, while walking over to the conference center, I bought a copy of the New York *Post*. The front page proclaimed: "CITY WANTS NAMES OF ALL AIDS CARRIERS. Dr. Joseph's new plan: City Health Commissioner Stephen Joseph will announce a new plan today to collect the names of everyone who tests positive for AIDS-virus infection." So here we go, I thought.

I began by setting the current context of the epidemic:

New York City recently recorded its 20,000th case of AIDS. Twenty thousand is a number of some significance, although of course HIV disease accounts for a much broader spectrum of illness.

It represents a degree of human suffering that we thought we would not see again from an infectious disease, reminding us that we are, to paraphrase Churchill, not at the beginning of the end, but only at the end of the beginning of AIDS.

It also represents an opportunity for us: to take stock of where we have been and where we are likely to go in the years ahead. Considering the widespread effect of AIDS upon the social, political, and economic life of New York, the city's experience with the epidemic is in many ways a foretelling of the future of AIDS for many other cities and countries of the world.

I then reviewed the past and projected future of AIDS in New York, concentrating on the increasing role of drug addiction.

Against this background, a panoply of changing public health and public policy issues faced New York. Early on, with little clinical intervention to offer HIV-infected people, our options for altering the course of the epidemic were educating the public and providing personal risk-reduction counselling and referrals for those whose behavior put them at risk of infection. We thus opposed mandatory testing and reporting of seropositives, and attempted only cautious contact tracing because we felt that these stances best helped us draw people at highest risk into our education and prevention system. From 1986 on, we rapidly, massively increased voluntary, confidential risk-reduction counselling and counselling-based HIV antibody testing citywide.

Many of our policies were controversial, necessarily so when trying to prevent a disease spread through behaviors associated with the most personal areas of human life, sexuality and drug use. Moralistic thinking placed obstacle after obstacle in the way of our condom initiative, AIDS prevention messages in the mass media, and needle exchange program. The Department of Health was denounced from press and pulpit for responding to imperatives of public health instead of presumptions of public morality. At times the science itself became the issue. Last summer much unhappiness influenced the reaction to our reduction of the estimates of HIV-infected New Yorkers from 400,000 to 200,000. But we performed our epidemiology and research without responding to political influence of any sort, and will continue to do so. . . .

But perhaps the major implication of the New York City experience concerns the public policy crossroads toward which we are rapidly moving. Science must drive policy; as the epidemic and our understanding of it evolve, our policies must change apace. Today we are fast approaching a time when we will have to rethink the wisdom and effectiveness of many of our present public policy stands.

It is only a matter of time before reliable published studies demonstrate the effectiveness of treatment for the asymptomatic HIV-infected person, or for preventing infection in an exposed person, or for reducing infectiousness of the person with HIV infection.

These changes in our capacity to prevent and treat infection will usher in a new era in which policies will shift toward a disease control approach to HIV infection along the lines of classic tuberculosis practices. Medically confidential counselling and testing will continue but become more aggressive and routine in high prevalence areas in all clinical settings. Within a confidential public health framework, reporting of seropositives, follow-up to assure adequate treatment, and more aggressive contact tracing will become standard public health applications for controlling HIV infection and illness. . . .

In this current time of transition, as at every other point in the pandemic, we will be best served by relying upon our constantly evolving knowledge, the willingness to engage in open debate around policies, and the flexibility to make such changes as we deem necessary.

The howls, shouted insults and obscenities, and sign waving had continued throughout my address, coming from a group of perhaps 100 to 150 protesters. As I finished (the electronic acoustics had been excellent, and I had not needed to raise my voice), I received a standing round of applause from the other several thousand people in the hall, though I am not at all certain whether it was for the content of my remarks or for my persistence in delivering them.

The reaction to my address was intense and immediate: rapid-fire questions from reporters in the halls, exclamations of support or opposition from conference attendees, and a request to appear at a press conference at the noontime break. The press conference was

another loud and tempestuous affair, with representatives of the gay
press shouting hostile statements masquerading as questions, along
with a strong interest by the general press in my call for mandatory
reporting of infection by physicians and hospitals and expanded
confidential counseling and testing and partner notification.

Corridor confrontations and street arguments continued throughout the day. When I returned to New York very early the next
morning, the media coverage was in full swing:

*New York Times:* HEALTH CHIEF URGES LISTING PEOPLE WITH THE
AIDS VIRUS

New York *Post:* BOOS AND CHEERS FOR AIDS PLAN

*Daily News:* AIDS SHOULD BE REPORTABLE, HEALTH COMMISH SAYS

*Newsday:* AIDS CONFERENCE DRAMA. OFFICIAL WANTS LIST KEPT OF
THE INFECTED

By the end of the week, the debate increased as activists re-
turning from Montreal voiced fears of anti-gay repression in the
guise of disease reporting. The major dailies ran editorials on the
subject: *Newsday* in opposition ("Naming Names. A provocative
new AIDS proposal stirs old fears"), and the *Post* ("Common Sense
on AIDS testing") and the *New York Times* ("The Case for Tracing
AIDS Partners") strongly in support.

The storm in Montreal and the subsequent tumult in New York
were really forerunners to an ongoing controversy that gathered
strength in the months that followed.

# Gracie Mansion

Right after the Montreal conference, ACT-UP organized a protest march which briefly blocked traffic on the Brooklyn Bridge during the morning rush hour, then moved to City Hall, and on to the nearby Health Department. They carried signs warning of abuses of mandatory reporting ("First You Don't Exist, Now You're on Joseph's List"), charged once again that the Mayor and the city were "ignoring" the AIDS problem, and displayed a poster (later to be put up as a bogus public service announcement in the subway cars) that showed my photograph and the words, "Deadlier than the Virus. Stephen C. Joseph, Commissioner of Health."

The mobilized gay community increased its pressures on the Mayor who, seeking a fourth term, was facing a difficult September 12 primary election. The Mayor announced that he was not certain whether he would support my Montreal proposals, and that he would convene a group of about thirty health care professionals, AIDS experts and advocates, within a week or so to advise him on the issue. This proposal, which was an aide's idea to deflect the pressure away from the Mayor, led to what I will always remember as the Saturday Morning Massacre.

The meeting was planned as a Saturday breakfast at Gracie Mansion, with twenty or so invited guests, including representatives of AIDS advocacy organizations (Mathilde Krim of the American Foundation for AIDS Research, Richard Dunne of Gay Men's Health Crisis, Jim Eigo of ACT-UP, Ron Johnson of the Minority Task Force on AIDS, and others), physicians and scientists prominent in AIDS work in the city. No other public health officials and no one from the state or federal public health establishments were to be present. The format was to be a response and discussion to a presentation by me of my proposals for expanded testing, contact tracing, and mandatory reporting, with the mayor presiding. It was quite clear ahead of time who was on the defensive, and who was to play the judge. I knew that I would face stiff prosecution from the advocates, but I based my hopes on receiving some open support from the health professionals, virtually all of whom assured me privately that they were in partial or full agreement with my positions.

As the days moved toward the breakfast, the state weighed in, and not to our assistance:

STATE NIXES CITY AIDS REPORT BID

State Health Commissioner David Axelrod yesterday torpedoed the city's request for mandatory reporting of the names of people infected with the AIDS virus.

Axelrod's opposition, as well as a tepid response from state legislative leaders, quashes a proposal by city Health Commissioner Stephen C. Joseph to use mandatory reporting as a tool to help locate and warn other people who may be infected with the HIV virus, which causes AIDS.

"The situation is evolving, but I see no reason for changing our policy at this time," said Axelrod, who has the authority to change the state's policy of keeping anonymous HIV records. "I think it would be premature to mandate reporting of HIV-infected persons."

Axelrod is unlikely to face pressure from the state Legislature to make the change, members of the Assembly and Senate health committees predicted. "I don't see any prospect for HIV-reporting legislation this session," said Assembly Health Committee Chairman Richard Gottfried (D-Manhattan).

An organized effort to kill the proposal emerged almost immediately after Joseph made the recommendation last week, in a speech at the Fifth International Conference on AIDS in Montreal. Forty physicians, public-health officials, and AIDS service groups signed a petition that they began circulating at the conference opposing mandatory reporting. . . .

"The suggestion that mandatory reporting will aid the populations most in need of services is a hollow promise, until the availability of therapeutic interventions, medical treatments, and primary health care is guaranteed," according to the statement, whose signatories include the American Foundation for AIDS Research and the Citizens Commission on AIDS.

Joseph said the prospect of expanded partner notification could be used to build the case for a dramatic expansion of medical services. "Sometimes the way you get a response is to turn up the heat on the stove," he said. . . .

Although he has been rebuffed by state officials in his call for mandatory reporting, Joseph vowed to step up voluntary partner notification, and will be asking that additional health department counselors be placed in clinics run by the city's 11 municipal hospitals.

*—Newsday,* June 14, 1989

and

CITY TO PRESS AIDS LIST

City Health Commissioner Stephen Joseph said yesterday he will keep pushing a plan to confidentially list the names of people who test positive for the AIDS virus despite opposition from key state officials and AIDS advocates.

"I'm going to continue to speak out on this issue and try to mobilize support," Joseph said. "I fully expect we will persevere and succeed."

*—Daily News,* June 15, 1989

I knew that the meeting was stacked against me, but I had no choice other than to make my best case and hope that the Mayor would support it. I knew from private discussion that both he and Stan Brezenoff agreed conceptually with my position, but I was also conscious that the realities of the approaching primary weighed heavily, especially as the Mayor drew more and more criticism from a gay community that had supported him strongly in previous elections.

The breakfast meeting was, from my perspective, a disaster. The advocates attacked strongly and persistently, and the medical experts shocked me by sitting almost completely silent. There was not a single statement of support for my position, except from Dr. Martin Cherkasky, emeritus president of the Montefiore Medical Center, and a friend and adviser to the Mayor.

At the end of the discussion, Ed Koch marched all of us downstairs to an impromptu press conference. (Gracie Mansion was besieged with media that morning.) To me it felt more like a public hanging than a press conference. The New York *Post* reported the meeting results accurately:

KOCH NIXES ANY LISTING OF AIDS CARRIERS

The city has rejected a proposal by its health commissioner that officials collect the names of those who test positive for the AIDS virus, Mayor Koch said yesterday.

Koch said the city needs to expand services for AIDS sufferers who come forward on their own before it tries to reach, through mandatory reporting, those sexual partners who don't know they may be infected.

Koch's unexpected announcement—after a closed-door meeting with more than a dozen AIDS activists and health officials—appeared to be a major defeat for Health Commissioner Stephen Joseph.

Joseph said two weeks ago at an international conference in Montreal that the names of AIDS-infected people should be reported confidentially to authorities and their contacts traced.

After the meeting yesterday, Joseph defended his statements in Montreal as "valid" opinions and said the Mayor did not rule out the possibility of mandatory reporting in the future.

"I didn't hear any future discussions foreclosed," Joseph said.

AIDS activists and many health officials had lambasted Joseph's idea—saying any infringement on anonymous testing would scare potentially infected people away from testing centers.

And, after yesterday's meeting, Koch concluded the city should continue the current system of anonymous testing.

"If there is to be a change, it can come only as a result of my agreeing to it," he said. "We haven't reached that."

Koch echoed the position of AIDS activists and said there are less controversial ways than contact tracing to reach out to New Yorkers who may be infected but don't know it.

He said he will urge counselors at drug treatment centers to get infected people to notify partners and place media ads encouraging people to come in for testing and treatment.

Koch did not rule out collecting names in the future, but activists left yesterday's meeting in Gracie Mansion convinced that will never happen.

"The Mayor came up with a way of repudiating Stephen Joseph's policy without publicly humiliating him," said Jim Eigo, a spokesman for the AIDS Coalition to Unleash Power.

Mathilde Krim, co-founder of the American Foundation for AIDS Research, said Joseph was the only one at the meeting defending his position.

"I don't like to call it a lesson, but I think he's thinking a little differently now," Krim said.

Jim and Mathilde were both wrong. I did feel publicly humiliated, and I wasn't thinking any differently about the public health importance of testing, contact tracing, and mandatory reporting.

In the hours after the meeting, I felt a strong urge to resign. This was the first time that the Mayor had publicly disassociated himself from my public health initiatives, and it was on a set of issues that I felt were vital to our responsibilities in the epidemic. Then I reasoned that Ed Koch had left the door open, and had also reassured me that he would not object to my continuing to speak out from the position I believed was correct. I decided to see it through, to push harder for counseling and testing and clinical services, to expand contact tracing wherever I could, and to accept that mandatory reporting would come on a future day, which I would try to hasten.

In August, Martin Cherkasky sent me an exchange of correspondence that he had with the Mayor in the weeks following the Gracie Mansion meeting. He urged the Mayor to support my proposals, to which the Mayor replied that before we considered a widespread policy change such as I had suggested, "we must reach out to the 40,000 or so drug addicts who have self-identified and seek to have them interviewed in order to trace their sex and drug partners. When we have finished, then we will have another meeting."

In my reply to Dr. Cherkasky, I said, "I find this the most bitter pill of the past three and a half years, and am haunted by the thoughts of the consequences of our dereliction of clinical and public health responsibility. I have, of course, not given up on finding some way to skin this cat."

After the Gracie Mansion meeting, the Mayor agreed to add significant additional AIDS funds into the executive budget, funds that had been previously been denied us in the closing rounds of the budget negotiations.

There was almost $5 million for expanded HIV primary care services in the Health and Hospitals Corporation, and about $1 million for additional counseling, testing, and public education through the Health Department. This additional funding, coming in a very tight budget year in which most programs and agencies were taking significant cuts, strengthened my conviction about the value of raising important policy issues forcefully, pursuing them aggressively, but also being able to argue from a reasoned position for their adoption, whether you won or lost.

I set the department to work, preparing a new public service advertising campaign that would encourage people at risk to be tested: "Take this simple AIDS test," the poster said, and then offered two checkoff boxes: "I want a fighting chance . . . I don't." It then went on to outline the benefits of early diagnosis and treatment.

With the additional funds, we began a program to put counselors in voluntary hospitals and drug treatment centers to encourage expanded testing in those settings. These workers were recruited, trained, and paid by the Health Department, but worked under the auspices of the assigned clinical facility. Funding constraints limited the number to about twenty, a small fraction of what was needed. We also issued a revision of the Guidelines on HIV Counseling and Testing that we had published in 1987 and sent to every physician practicing in the city; in the revision we gave much more importance to the need for the physician to assure partner notification, and of the Health Department's willingness to help. We also suggested that each physician might want to keep a confidential list in his own records of his HIV-infected patients.

Meanwhile, on September 12, Ed Koch was decisively defeated in the Democratic mayoral primary election by David Dinkins. The gay community voted heavily for a change at City Hall.

I continued to speak and write in support of my Montreal proposals, especially before groups concerned with minority and women's health issues.

But the most tangible opportunity for "skinning the cat" came from an unlikely direction: the Medical Examiner's Office, a quasi-independent agency that reported in theory but not in practice to the Health Commissioner. When the Mayor fired Dr. Elliott Gross, the previous Medical Examiner, he set up an advisory committee to find a replacement and oversee the office on his behalf.

The Mayor appointed Martin Cherkasky as chairman. I was one of the other five committee members. We recruited Dr. Charles Hirsch, who had one of the strongest reputations in the country as a forensic pathologist of competence, integrity, and innovation. I soon learned that he was as eager as I to press ahead on all possible fronts to combat the epidemic.

Since the Medical Examiner has jurisdiction over all bodies of persons who have died of drug-related causes, victims of violence, and unidentified bodies, we were sure that a high proportion of M.E. cases were HIV-positive. Dr. Gross had never been very forthcoming about AIDS-related research, but Dr. Hirsch quickly made clear that his position was the opposite.

A few rapidly carried out studies showed that HIV prevalence among the 10,000 M.E. autopsies annually was even higher than expected, as high as 40 percent of all autopsies in one series. Chuck Hirsch and I came up with a two-stage proposal, which we planned to present first to the Cherkasky committee and then to the Mayor.

In stage one, the Medical Examiner would begin routine HIV-antibody testing of all corpses that came to him. This would provide valuable information regarding AIDS and drug addiction. The information would be reported only statistically to the Health Department; personal identification would remain confidential.

In stage two, the Health Department would train and assign HIV counselors to the Medical Examiner's Office. These counselors, acting under the administration of the M.E. Office, would notify spouses and steady sexual partners of those HIV-positive deceased persons whose medical records did not indicate a prior diagnosis of HIV illness (that is, where there was no reasonable cause to expect that the partner already knew of the risk). Again, the personally identifying information would be kept by the Medical Examiner, and not turned over to Health Department records.

Under this plan, we would counter the charge (sure to be made by AIDS advocates and civil libertarians) that we were trying to sneak mandatory reporting in the back door. It seemed inconceivable to us that there could be any serious objection to warning the partner of a deceased individual, a partner who would have no other way of learning of the risk. And, further, it would be a very high-yield operation; Dr. Hirsch estimated we would find more than a thousand unsuspected cases a year.

Dr. Cherkasky was enthusiastic; we got the plan through the oversight committee in late November without significant opposition. Best of all, the Mayor was strongly supportive of both stages, and gave us the go-ahead, asking only that we inform (not ask permission, but inform) the Dinkins transition staff that we were starting the program.

Stage one went into operation. The results were impressive, with almost 20 percent of all autopsies in the first year recording a positive HIV test. Unfortunately, stage two, which would have yielded important and direct benefits to the unsuspecting living, was shelved by the new Mayor, at the urging of AIDS advocacy groups, whose reasoning in this instance I find unfathomable and directly harmful to the well-being of specific individuals (mostly minority women) and to the community at large.

I knew I would be leaving my position with the advent of the

Dinkins administration; the new Mayor had taken strong positions opposite to mine on needle exchange, and on the testing-tracing-and-reporting issue. In mid-December I testified before the New York State Assembly Committee on Health's Task Force on AIDS. This was to be my last formal statement on these issues as commissioner. I drew together the threads connecting confidentiality, the duty to warn, and the Montreal proposals. I began by noting that the critically important law that became effective on February 1, 1989 set out parameters for HIV testing, mandated confidentiality of HIV-related information and records, and permitted disclosure of the information in certain circumstances. It also permitted physicians to disclose confidential HIV information to a contact whom the physician reasonably believed to be at risk when the patient refused to notify the contact.

Since passage of the law, I noted we had entered a new stage of the epidemic:

> The federal Centers for Disease Control's recommendation that all HIV-infected persons be medically evaluated every six months, and other studies that have shown the benefit of early diagnosis of HIV infection and early access and entry into treatment for earlier forms of HIV illness and even asymptomatic infection, have increased the importance of even more vigorously offering widespread counseling and HIV antibody testing.

> I strongly believe that physicians and health care institutions should be required to offer counseling and testing to all pregnant women because of the very high rates of perinatal transmission in the city and the state.

> When a serious exposure presenting a substantial risk of HIV infection occurs to public servants protecting society on a first-response basis, they should have as much information as possible. [State law] should be amended to authorize a court to order HIV-related testing, without consent, upon a showing that a police officer, fire fighter, or emergency health care worker is at "significant risk of HIV infection as a result of exposure to" the person to be tested. The standards of evidence

and proof should be the same as those high standards now required to obtain a court ordered disclosure of confidential HIV-related information. . . .

The physician's so-called permission to warn has not worked. There have been no referrals to the New York City Department of Health by physicians since enactment of the law. Discussions with practicing physicians suggest that the physicians themselves are not notifying contacts either, but, if anything, are suggesting that patients tell partners or refer partners to the Health Department. Before the law was enacted, our reading of New York common law was that the physician had a duty to warn; Section 2782(4) was specifically crafted to replace that duty with permission. It now ought to be redrafted to require that the physician either ensure the patient has notified known contacts of risk, or notify such contacts or the Health Department; a "duty to have warned" must ensure that people at risk are warned.

I went on to say that medicine's increasing capacity to prevent and treat HIV infection obliged us to take more vigorous infection control measures because we have clear health benefits to offer those who are infected. Early diagnosis of infection and illness benefits both society and the individual. Medicine's ability to increase the quality and length of life of HIV-infected persons makes a stronger case for accepted public health measures for case finding. I believe that AIDS policies, buttressed by the AIDS confidentiality law, should shift to a disease control approach to HIV infection along the lines of classic tuberculosis practices. I also argued that that mandatory but confidential public health reporting of seropositive people was an inevitable development and went on to say:

Today's hearing is an opportunity not only to continue shaping a confidentiality law that will support this critical public health measure, but to begin considering the legislative implications of public health reporting of seropositives. Otherwise we will lose our new opportunities to develop the fully effective programs, especially availability of massively expanded clinical and social services, that are so vital. . . .

The legislators listened politely, and asked few questions. Nothing was done.

# 8

## *The Needle Exchange*

It's genocide, pure and simple. . . . When the first needle is given out by Dr. Joseph, he ought to be indicted and arrested for murder and drug distribution.

—City Councilman Hilton Clark,
representing central Harlem

At the press conference accompanying my swearing-in as Commissioner of Health on May 1, 1986, the first question I was asked was, "There are reports that the radioactive cloud emanating from the Chernobyl disaster is drifting toward New York. Is the city in any danger?" The second question was, "Your predecessor favored giving clean needles to drug addicts to prevent the spread of AIDS. What is your position?"

The first question was easily dispensed with: No New York cloud. No fallout. No danger. But the second was to become an ongoing battle and an endless series of obstacles that lasted beyond the final day of my tenure, almost four years later.

Even in my relative state of innocence in dealing with the New York media, I knew that needle exchange would be a contentious issue. I tried to keep my reply measured: "Anything that might help in the AIDS epidemic should be considered. I'm in favor of trying a small-scale experiment by which to study the question of whether the distribution of clean needles would do good, or for that matter, do harm."

From that day forward, the needle exchange issue would be a dominant theme in my life. Needle exchange would become a national issue, polarize the city, lead to my being labeled a racist, genocidal, drug-pushing murderer, and contribute to Ed Koch's loss in his bid for a fourth term as Mayor of the City of New York.

As a specific measure to prevent blood-to-blood transmission of HIV among heroin addicts, sterile injection equipment was already being provided to addicts in several Western European cities, either as a legally sanctioned program or as an act of civil disobedience by physicians or advocates for drug abusers.

A variety of programs in the United Kingdom (in London, Liverpool, Edinburgh, Glasgow), New Zealand, Australia, the Netherlands, and Sweden had presented suggestive but fragmented evidence that the availability of clean equipment decreased needle sharing by addicts, did not increase needle use or drug injection, and might stabilize transmission rates of HIV among groups of addicts.

Opponents of needle exchange claimed that sharing injection equipment was part of the "culture of drug use," that addicts were unreliable as both research subjects and service clients, and that providing injection equipment lent an aura of legitimacy and thus promoted intravenous drug use. Law enforcement officials, in particular, argued that the criminalization of drug paraphernalia aided successful drug arrests and prosecutions.

In the United States, the issue was moot in the thirty-nine states where possession of drug-injecting equipment required no medical prescription, and where possession of such equipment was not illegal. Only eleven states and the District of Columbia restricted possession of needles and syringes. These included many of the jurisdictions where intravenous drug abuse was most intense: California, District of Columbia, Illinois, Massachusetts, New Jersey, New York, Pennsylvania. Nowhere in the nation, however, not even in those states where possession of injection equipment was legal, did a proactive public health program make needles readily available as a deliberate measure to slow AIDS transmission.

In mid-August 1985, my predecessor as Health Commissioner, Dr. David Sencer, had sent a memo to Mayor Koch proposing that he support a change in state law to remove the prohibition against possessing injection equipment without medical prescription. The

Mayor circulated the memo to the district attorneys of the five boroughs, all of whom strongly opposed the idea. They were joined by a virtually unanimous chorus of rejection among law enforcement officials and city politicians. The trial balloon never got off the ground.

However, the New York Bar Association's Committee on Medicine and the Law began a formal study of the question. They issued a report in May 1986 recommending that in response to the epidemic the state legalize the purchase of hypodermic needles and syringes without a prescription. Their sober and carefully drawn report was virtually ignored in the debates that followed. When New York State Assemblyman Richard Gottfried (later Chairman of the Assembly Health Committee) proposed a bill in the spring of 1987 that would legalize over-the-counter sales, he was unable to find a single cosponsor.

As I considered the issue in May 1986, I thought it self-evident that:

- there was urgent need to take all feasible preventive action to reduce needle transmission of HIV;
- pious exhortations for "universal drug treatment" or even "treatment on demand" for addicts were unlikely to be matched by actual major increases in drug treatment capacity, at least in the short run of relevance to the AIDS epidemic;
- there was zero chance of a change in state law regarding needle possession, and even such a change would not necessarily reach those most at risk or posing the greatest risk to others;
- any efforts to move in this direction would meet intense political opposition and attract few allies.

I thought that the best course was to push directly for a Health Department program exchanging sterile for unsterile needles and syringes as a public health measure, hoping to demonstrate the success of this approach on a small scale, and then pressing for wider authorization. I also felt that our knowledge was inadequate in this field, and that a small pilot research program might yield important details. I personally believed strongly that needle exchange was an appropriate measure that would do far more good than any harm it might possibly cause, and that it was fully justified given the critical situation.

I also knew that sufficient scientific data did not exist to substantiate that belief firmly, and hoped that a successful pilot program would give us the tools we needed to expand. Against this, of course, was the realization that a limited experiment would consume several years of precious time, pushing further off into the future the effective reduction of AIDS transmission.

That sort of difficult choice is not unusual in public health. In this instance it was easy to make the choice, since the go-for-it-all legislative approach had absolutely no chance of winning approval at this stage. Further, the research approach had an appealingly useful loophole to it.

It is true that state law authorizes penalties for illegal possession of injection equipment, and thus a direct approach to either needle distribution or a change in the law would have to overcome the resistance of law enforcement, judicial, and legislative forces as well as broad-based political opinion. In other words, formidable forces were arrayed on the side of criminal penalties for possession.

Yet the field of public health was not without resources of its own. It is the state Health Commissioner who has the power to define who may legally possess needles and syringes. The state's public health law makes it unlawful to sell or furnish hypodermic needles or syringes except to persons with a written prescription or persons who have been authorized by the (state) Commissioner of Health.

The strategy we adopted, then, involved an attempt to persuade Dr. David Axelrod to grant an exemption to the law for a "class of persons" in New York City, who would become research subjects in a pilot study to be carried out by the city Department of Health. This would, we thought, bypass legal and formal political obstacles and allow us to get on with the urgent task at hand. In actuality, gaining state approval to the project was to consume more than two years—two years that set us ever further behind the epidemic, and allowed unchecked increase of HIV infections.

I made no secret of my intention to devise some sort of needle exchange program, and as this became generally known the opposition grew widespread and vociferous. I had the support of the Mayor. Although I knew he was skeptical, he was willing to let me try, and even gave me cautious but explicit public support. In this he was alone among all political figures in the city.

Public health officials around the country showed interest and support, but no one seemed to be able to overcome community opposition to needle exchange. Dr. Molly Coye, the New Jersey Health Commissioner, announced in the summer of 1986 that she would authorize a pilot program in that state, but quickly had to withdraw her plans in the face of overwhelming legislative hostility —hostility that seemingly ignored the fact that New Jersey had the clearest IV drug-driven AIDS profile in the nation.

Given the Mayor's willingness to provide me all the rope I wanted with which to hang myself, I thought we could get a program moving. The key element was to get David Axelrod to clear our path. We began discussions with the state Health Department on what kind of program would be mutually acceptable.

After months of back and forth, we suddenly sensed daylight: In response to the release of a National Academy of Sciences report saying, "It is time to begin experimenting with public policy to encourage the use of sterile needles and syringes by removing legal and administrative barriers to their possession and use," Dr. Axelrod issued a statement saying: "I think it is worthwhile to consider, as the National Academy has suggested, limited trials that can be controlled to determine whether or not there is any effect on the transmission of the AIDS virus in the intravenous drug population."

Though Dr. Axelrod's support was half-hearted at best, I thought we had enough to push ahead with, and I used a local Sunday morning television program to announce that we had "preliminary agreement between the Mayor and the state Health Commissioner to proceed with the development of such a project," a somewhat generous but not grossly inaccurate interpretation of the facts. Trying to achieve as much momentum as possible, I added (totally unrealistically, as it turned out): "We are hopeful that we can get something off the ground in the next couple of months."

That set the cat among the pigeons, and reaction was swift from all corners. David Axelrod made it clear that we would have to present a research design that would jump through a whole set of scientific hoops and snares. City Council and other political figures rushed to condemn the idea as "sending a mixed message on drugs." Media conservatives such as the *Daily News*'s Raymond Coffey shrilled, "Free Needles and Condoms? It's Madness!" Sterling Johnson, Jr., the city's special narcotics prosecutor, likened the plan to "having city-run shooting galleries." Johnson, a plain-speaking, street-tough black prosecutor with strong credibility, became one of our most formidable opponents in the rising debate, which quickly took on a racial context as black politicians and community leaders condemned the idea as being specially aimed at black drug addicts.

Just how much this issue could polarize discussion and debate was soon seen at one of the Mayor's town meetings, open forums that he held around the city (130 in his twelve-year tenure). The Mayor habitually took along a group of his commissioners and had them respond to specific questions that were asked related to their areas of responsibility.

Police Commissioner Ben Ward and I attended such a meeting in largely black East New York, a Brooklyn neighborhood with a severe drug problem. During a momentary lull in the discussion, the Mayor, who would instigate controversy if it lagged, said to the virtually 100 percent black audience, "You've heard about this idea of giving clean needles to addicts to stop AIDS. Here are my Police Commissioner and my Health Commissioner; one is against it and the other is for it. Why don't they each make their case to you, and then you tell them what you think."

Seldom have I felt more like the fish in the barrel, and the audience let us know clearly how they felt even before we began. Ben Ward went first. He laid out the "mixed messages" and "promotion of drug abuse" arguments. Then he launched into a diatribe against the program as racial injustice—Ben is black—invoking the powerful ghosts of the Tuskegee experiment and suggesting that we (I, actually) were again preparing to use black people as guinea pigs. He turned to me and said: "If you want to do needle exchange, why don't you go up to Scarsdale and do it there?"

After that it hardly mattered what I said in rebuttal. I felt fortunate to get out of the hall with my shirt on.

Within a day or so, I had a letter from Commissioner Ward:

I want to take this opportunity after some review of my remarks the other night, to apologize for the manner in which I disagreed with your recommendations concerning "clean needles" for drug addicts.

I still disagree with your recommendation; however, upon reflection I believe I could have disagreed in a more "agreeable manner." Please accept my apologies, nothing personal was intended. Sincerely, Ben.

I wrote back:

Thank you for your letter of December 3. It was very much appreciated, though no apology was needed, and no offense was taken. I believe that colleagues can, and should, disagree vigorously. I know that we share the same objectives here: 1) do nothing to worsen the drug problem, 2) do everything possible to slow the spread of AIDS. I am most interested in working together to find the best way through this thicket. . . .

The AIDS crisis is of dimensions that are only beginning to be grasped. None of us enjoys "thinking the unthinkable," but we are searching for every avenue that might assist. With best regards, I remain, Sincerely yours, Steve.

Commissioner Ward remained personally and publicly opposed to the project, but he was always as good as his word to work together productively. From the day we finally got the needle exchange going, we never once had a single incident of police harassment of the addicts enrolled in the program, and the Police Department helped explain our intentions to the local precincts.

In spite of the public spotlight, however, our greatest obstacle at this stage was the state Health Department. Safely insulated in Albany, they led us on a not-so-merry chase toward what we hoped would be approval of our research design.

We faced a major tactical problem. If we designed a project large enough to yield statistically significant answers to the research questions, we would need several thousand participants. Such a large project would infuriate the opposition who might then gather enough strength to kill it. On the other hand, a smaller, less conspicuous, scientifically weaker project would be less likely to be acceptable on methodologic grounds to Dr. Axelrod.

We were hooked on the horns of a dilemma. The state rejected our first plan as being too large and then the revision as too small.

I was now more determined than ever to succeed with a needle exchange demonstration, both for what it might offer New York and because I was convinced that if we gave up here, no other jurisdiction would be able to overcome the cumulative history of opposition and give a reading on this critical question, a reading based on experience rather than prejudice.

Throughout the summer and fall of 1987, we redoubled our efforts to come to agreement with the state on a program design that would be acceptable. This was perhaps made easier because the din of public opposition had muted, since most people assumed the idea was dead.

By December 1987, we had made substantial progress. There were hints from Albany that Dr. Axelrod was reconsidering his long-standing opposition. Once again, we were close to achieving our objective, and once again an event occurred to threaten our efforts.

In early January 1988, the issue was nearly taken out of our hands. In an attempt to force an end to the bureaucratic and political delays, a community service group known as ADAPT (the Association for Drug Abuse Prevention and Treatment) announced it would begin to distribute needles and syringes to addicts in New York City as an act of civil disobedience.

ADAPT, whose major source of financial support was grant funds from the Department of Health, was well-known to me. The group was probably the most effective in the city at working with addicts on the street, getting them into drug treatment, and lobbying for health and social services. I had met with ADAPT's president, Yolanda Serrano, and her board members on several occasions, and admired their work.

Yolanda and company had run out of patience, and were prepared
to face prosecution and the loss of financing and tax-exempt status
to, as she put it, "protect the public and save lives."

Both my sympathies and my own frustrations were with ADAPT.
However, I felt certain that their civil disobedience in the already
highly charged setting would be the kiss of death for needle exchange. Both city and state governments would have to come down
hard on ADAPT, and public opinion was definitely against the idea.
More substantively, an "uncontrolled" random distribution of needles would lose us the opportunity to try to gather persuasive data
on the question.

In this tight spot, the Mayor played his cards to strengthen, rather
than weaken, my hand. Under a headline of ED: I'LL BUST CLEAN
NEEDLE TEAM, the New York *Post* reported:

Mayor Koch yesterday threatened to arrest activists caught
handing out free needles to drug addicts—even though he's
"supportive" of their cause. The Mayor expressed sympathy for
ADAPT, a private drug-abuse agency which wants to help halt
the spread of AIDS by distributing clean needles—in violation
of state law. Koch said, "They will be arrested if they violate
the law. . . . Even if I am for this, we will not allow people to
break the law with impunity." Koch lashed State Health Commissioner David Axelrod and the Legislature for nixing experimental projects to hand out clean needles. The mayor said he
supports a program proposed by city Health Commissioner
Stephen Joseph to give needles to limited groups of addicts.
"The Legislature was against it, the DA's were against it," and
Axelrod rejected a similar proposal, Koch said.

I telephoned Yolanda, reassured her of my support for ADAPT's
goals, tried to convey the risks should they proceed illegally, and
then said flatly that if they did proceed I was sure that the police
would arrest them and that, more to the point, I would take whatever steps I could to withdraw our financial support of the organization immediately.

That pulled the situation back from the brink. ADAPT dropped their plans for street distribution, and we continued what was a mutually supportive partnership. When we were finally able to begin needle exchange, we depended on ADAPT's street outreach capability for a large share of our recruitment of program clients.

The ADAPT threat had another important result: it smoked out the first public comment on needle exchange from the Governor, who was reported in the *New York Times* as saying, despite his former position of opposition to the idea, "But I have an open mind . . . (the issue has been) tormenting me—its very, very difficult." Was this a straw in the wind?

The breakthrough came swiftly now. Within three weeks of the ADAPT incident, the *New York Times* Albany capital reporter called to tell me that the next day a Sunday story, ADDICTS TO GET NEEDLES IN PLAN TO CURB AIDS, would run:

> The Cuomo administration, reversing an earlier stand, will let New York City distribute clean needles to hundreds of drug addicts as part of an experiment to reduce the spread of AIDS, officials familiar with the administration's thinking said today.

A follow-up article made the political point clearly:

> Which is more of a threat to New York today, the spread of heroin addiction or the spread of AIDS? And to the Cuomo administration, it presented a politically dangerous choice: being seen as soft on drugs or being seen as slow and ineffective in combating AIDS. In the end, officials said, new data on AIDS made it clear to the Cuomo administration that, whatever the other dangers, it must now try new strategies to fight the disease. As a result, the state Health Commissioner, Dr. David Axelrod, reversed two years of opposition to the experiment.

Once again it looked as if the key step was in sight. Once again the Mayor endorsed the idea—and left no doubt whose neck was in the noose: "I am pleased that Dr. Stephen Joseph's proposal will be given an opportunity to be tried, and I hope it's successful. If it is, it will save lives. If it is not, we'll end it."

It quickly became clear, however, that the state was not approving any *specific* program, just indicating in general its willingness to go along with one if a satisfactory methodology could be agreed upon. Were we really any further ahead?

Whether we were or not, hostile reaction was not slow in coming. On the same day that the *New York Times* story ran, John Cardinal O'Connor said after Mass at Saint Patrick's Cathedral: "It drags down the standards of all society. . . . It is an act born of desperation." The Reverend Calvin Butts, pastor of the Abyssinian Baptist Church in Harlem said, "I am not in favor of cooperating with evil. . . . If we give out needles now . . . the next step will be to legalize crack and heroin." Special narcotics prosecutor Sterling Johnson, Jr., suggested that I would be guilty of felony action if the program actually began, and threatened to arrest and prosecute Dr. Axelrod and me; this was bluster on his part, since he must have known that the law gave us the authority to act, but his comments inflamed the situation still further.

We again redoubled our efforts to design a program plan that would meet with state approval for scientific validity—and public debate and criticism redoubled. I made numerous presentations and engaged in seemingly endless debate about the idea on television, in newspaper columns, and in meetings with medical and other professional groups, focusing on meetings particularly with black physicians, where the hottest criticism was coming from.

On February 19, 1988, I received formal notice from Dr. Axelrod that the state would move forward. His letter laid out the specific elements of a scientific protocol that would have to be agreed upon before final approval would be given. A mild-sounding sentence added a further hurdle for us to surmount: "To ensure the cooperation of the relevant law enforcement agencies, I would appreciate your providing us with documentation of the participation of the Mayor's Criminal Justice Coordinator, the Police Commissioner, and the Special Assistant District Attorney For Narcotics Enforcement."

The first two could be enlisted, but the "participation" of Sterling

Johnson, Jr., who was continuing to threaten Axelrod and me with arrest if we proceeded, was not in the cards. I chose an alternative strategy, which proved effective in the end: to ask the city's Corporation Counsel Peter Zimroth to give us a legal opinion about conducting a needle exchange under Dr. Axelrod's research authority, and the indemnity from prosecution of myself and Health Department staff. It took some more precious time, but on July 29, Peter Zimroth wrote me his opinion that the study was legal.

We could not have achieved this critical advance, of course, without the steady support of the Mayor, whose influence with his own Police Commissioner, Criminal Justice Coordinator, and Corporation Counsel was considerable. Ed Koch also agreed to budget $250,000 to fund the program if and when it was approved; that money remained protected until it was used in the following year, despite competing demands in what became a very tight budget. Despite the vocal opposition of the city's entire black political leadership, the Mayor stood by us in proceeding with what *Time* magazine called "the lesser of two evils." Harlem Congressman Charles Rangel, Chairman of the House Select Committee on Narcotics Abuse and Control, called the program "A quick fix . . . I am not prepared to condone, even on an experimental basis, handing clean needles to addicts in exchange for used ones."

With the legal hurdles cleared, the pace toward program approval picked up and on August 12 the *New York Times* accurately reported that we would be distributing needles to 200 addicts with the approval of state health officials. This would be the first time a government agency in the country had distributed needles. The *Times* quoted Sterling Johnson, Jr., the city's special narcotics prosecutor: "What a terrible signal this sends in the war on drugs." Johnson conceded the experiment was legal but noted the high drug use among minorities and said the plan had "racist implications."

This small pilot needle exchange study was from its inception constrained by the hostile realities of New York City. We were to be limited to only a handful of working sites and to a very small number of registrants even though we knew from what the developers of analogous programs in other countries told us that it was important to make the activity "user friendly," to minimize the inconveniences and administrative and legal obstacles that the drug addict had to surmount in order to participate in the program.

Some of the other programs were uncontrolled giveaways or simple exchanges of dirty needles for clean. Our objective, however, was to try to learn more about the transaction in as disciplined and scientific a fashion as possible: what the motivations, behaviors, and therapeutic possibilities were, and what the HIV-infection status of program participants was. Further, we were determined to place the needle exchange itself in a broader preventive and therapeutic context, combining exchange with education about AIDS risk reduction, and with efforts to get addicts off drugs and into treatment.

The project design finally agreed upon looked like this: 400 enrollees—200 in the test group and 200 controls. They had to be referred to us by an existing drug treatment program, where they had either been admitted but placed on a waiting list, or rejected because the drug treatment program had no room for them. Those desiring to participate in needle exchange "until a spot opened up for them in drug treatment" would be randomly assigned to either the test or control group. Participants would receive a physical examination (including examination for needle tracks to prove that they were indeed intravenous drug users), tests for syphilis, tuberculosis, hepatitis B, and counseling and testing for HIV infection. All participants would receive education on HIV risk reduction (sexual as well as drug-related), condoms, bleach, sterile water, cotton and bottle-cap cooker, active assistance in gaining entrance to drug treatment (which would take precedence over continuing provision of needles), and assistance in connecting with health and social services.

The only difference between test and control groups would be that the test participants would be given a needle and syringe, which they could bring back at any time to the program and exchange for another set. Only one set would be provided at a time, and subjects who did not return the set on several occasions would be dropped.

The needles and syringes were imprinted with a special Health Department logo that identified them as part of the project, and were contained in a puncture-proof metal container issued to each test subject. Under state regulations, registered participants who were found with the specially marked equipment were not in violation of the paraphernalia law. Participants had, however, no legal immunity from laws regarding drug possession, commission of any other offense, or possession of any needle and syringe except the specially marked ones.

Registered participants carried a laminated photo identification card, with a code number instead of their name. If picked up by the police while having a Health Department-marked syringe, the participant was to show the ID, whereupon the police would call a needle exchange emergency telephone number where the specific individual's actual participation in the program could be confirmed. (Though seemingly cumbersome, this system of identity confirmation worked quite well; the five times the police called for verification, the individuals were released uneventfully).

On each visit for needle exchange, counseling and risk-reduction education was repeated, and efforts were made to find an available drug treatment program for the client.

As progress toward the actual start-up of the program gathered steam, so too did the virulence of the opposition.

The public criticism fell into four major categories: first, needle exchange not only would not work, but would abet and promote further drug abuse (it did not seem to bother those making this argument that there was not a shred of evidence to back it up, and quite a bit of experience from the European programs to the contrary).

Second, the program was being developed in secret, as a kind of conspiracy (this, even though every facet of the needle exchange had been debated intensely in meetings large and small, and with a vengeance in the media, for almost two years).

Third, needle exchange was a preliminary step to the legalization of heroin and cocaine (even though the Mayor and I on every possible occasion voiced our opposition to legalization of drugs and drug use).

Fourth, this program was overtly and deliberately aimed with hostile intent at black New Yorkers. This argument struck a particularly raw nerve, and was deliberately used by the program's opponents to discredit it and its proponents.

One of the most vicious advocates of the "racist conspiracy" arguments was Harlem City Councilman Hilton Clark, who began by sending the Mayor and me a letter accusing us of "cynically" abusing blacks: "You're telling us that it is all right for Black people to use heroin to kill themselves, and that it is all right to rob from other Blacks to maintain a heroin habit."

More disturbing was the almost total opposition of responsible black leaders, including the newly formed Black Leadership Commission on AIDS, a distinguished group which gave some hope to the possibility of mobilizing black community action against AIDS. The commission regrettably joined the chorus of absurd apocalyptic predictions. A group letter signed by prominent black New York congressmen and medical leaders echoed the hyperbole: "All of this is being done in the name of public health, but it would have disastrous public health consequences. It is obvious that such a program would lead to a breakdown of law and order in minority group communities in New York City and to wholesale destruction of these people."

The City Council's Minority Caucus added their anger, calling the proposal "beyond reason." Caucus member Wendell Foster labeled the program, "Planned assassination in the Black community. It's a damnable, intolerable, unforgivable project."

But it was the city's black weekly newspaper, the *Amsterdam News*, that brought the race-baiting to its height, and that first overtly linked needle exchange with the upcoming mayoral campaign. After a series of articles and editorials opposing the program, editor-in-chief Wilbert Tatum wrote the following piece. Mr. Tatum's diatribe, and my response, are perhaps the most complete statements of the opposing points of view on needle exchange in New York City, and illustrate the inability of the two sides to have a rational discussion. For that reason, they are reprinted here in full:

KOCH MUST RESIGN

The utter arrogance of Edward I. Koch and his Commissioner

of Health, Stephen Joseph, who have had the audacity to impose their flawed wisdom in a situation so fraught with danger that anyone but a fool can see it. These two less than brilliant men have decided to go ahead with what they refer to as a Needle Exchange Program.

These guys aren't talking about the kinds of needles you sew with. They are talking about the kinds of needles you use to shoot some substance into your veins. They are talking about exchanging clean needles for dirty needles with 200 of New York's 200,000 heroin-addicted citizens. They say that this will prevent, or help to prevent, the spread of AIDS. Thus, in the name of AIDS therapy, and on the backs of the Black and Latino communities, these two "hopelessly white" men have unilaterally decided what is best for these communities, and will (they tell everybody) begin to distribute these needles legally in order that the heroin addicts can inject with cleanliness an illegal substance that is bought from a person or persons that Koch wants to have executed by the State if they kill a cop while under the influence or committing a crime in order to buy more drugs (illegally) to shoot up with the clean needles that were bought with our tax dollars. Is this stupid, or what? Koch and Joseph will do this, they say, whether the community wants it or not, and they'll put the centers for distribution precisely where they want them, just as soon as they have told the communities where they'll go. This attitude is entirely consistent with Koch's attitude about minorities, as well as his attitude about the communities he is supposed to be serving as mayor.

It is not like Joseph and Koch didn't try to get approval, or at least silent tolerance of this outrage. They went to everybody trying to sell this shaky bill of goods. Their entreaties were rejected out of hand by Dr. James Curtis, head of the psychiatric unit at Harlem Hospital; by Dr. Phyllis Harrison-Ross, director of the community mental health program at Metropolitan Hospital; and by Dr. Beny Prim, himself a legend in the war against drugs and director of one of the largest and most effective drug treatment programs in the nation. These physicians have already forgotten more than Koch or Joseph ever knew about drug treatment therapy. Besides, they not only come in contact with addicts on a daily basis, they're not afraid to touch them. The addicts are not an abstraction to them. To these dedicated physicians, they are sick human beings who can be helped and must be saved.

The opposition to the idiocy of this needle exchange program doesn't stop with these physicians. The Black and Hispanic Caucus of the City Council is unanimously opposed to it, and have demanded that the Mayor cancel the program. City Council Member Hilton Clark, who represents central Harlem went even further: He said that, "When the first needle is given out by Dr. Joseph, he ought to be indicted and arrested for murder and drug distribution."

New York City's entire congressional delegation, including Congressman Charles B. Rangel, head of the House Select Sub-Committee on Drug and Substance Abuse, are against the program. The newly formed New York City Black Commission on AIDS voted unanimously to reject the program following a presentation by Dr. Joseph three short weeks ago. It seems that everybody, including the editors of the Daily News and New York Newsday are against the Needle Exchange Program. Why, then, this dogmatic approach to something that immediately affects communities with which both Koch and Joseph are unfamiliar? This is so hard to answer. Yet, the simplest reason, especially given the massive corruption of city officials in the Koch administration, is that somebody has a brother in the needle business. It is just as good an answer as any. It simply doesn't make any sense.

What is probably more likely is that Koch wants once more to let Blacks and Latinos know who's boss in this town, and that he can do whatever the hell he wants and get away with it.

What Koch is saying is: Your clergy doesn't matter. Your politicians don't matter. Your medical community sucks wind. Your community leaders are cowards, and you Blacks and Latinos are dumb as hell. I will do precisely what I want, 'cause I am the mayor.

For this kind of incredible arrogance, insensitivity and down-right fatal reasoning, KOCH MUST RESIGN OR BE RE-MOVED.

I wrote back to Mr. Tatum a reply which he never saw fit to publish:

Your recent editorial (November 5, 1988) opposing the Health Department's needle exchange study was inaccurate in the extreme. And, worse, it trivialized the terrible and all-too-real circumstances that compel us to study needle exchange.

The AIDS epidemic is bearing down on the city's minority communities like a downhill runaway locomotive. AIDS is already the number-one killer of Black men and women aged 25 to 44, and the third largest overall killer of Blacks in New York City. And since I last wrote you, on October 7 (nb two months earlier), more than 470 new cases have been reported—that's more than 15 cases every day—and fully two-thirds of those new cases (that's ten every day) have been among Blacks or Hispanics. Of 17 new AIDS cases among children, 15 are Black or Hispanic.

The unfortunate truth is that these numbers grow larger, month-by-month and year-by-year, and will keep growing unless we do everything in our power to stop the spread of AIDS from IV drug user to other IV drug users, and from IV drug users to their sex partners and unborn children.

It is time to face the hard reality that there are 200,000 IV drug users here, that some 100,000 are already infected with the AIDS virus, and that there is only room enough in treatment for 35,000. We must get more drug treatment on line quickly—that's the number-one priority! But at the same time we must not abandon the majority of IV drug users who will remain outside of treatment for the foreseeable future, as well as their sex partners and their babies, to the high probability of infection, illness, and death from the AIDS virus. That, simply, is why we must try needle exchange: It has been tried successfully elsewhere, and may well be able to save lives here.

Your claim that "everybody, including the editors of . . . New York Newsday" opposes the study is bogus, when, in fact, Newsday has staunchly and repeatedly endorsed it.

And listing only those who oppose the study, while pointedly omitting any mention of the many health and drug treatment experts in favor, distorts the issue. You should include the opinions of the Surgeon General, the National Academy of Sciences/Institute of Medicine Task Force on AIDS, the American Public Health Association, the New York County Medical Society, the Committee on Medicine and the Law of the Association of the Bar of the City of New York, the World Health Organization, the New York State Committee of Methadone Program Administrators, and many of the nation's leading drug treatment and public health experts, who, among others, call for exploring the availability of sterile injection equipment.

Your allegation that the study targets Blacks and Hispanics is utterly false. The study in no way targets minorities, but does target intravenous drug users, in particular those IV drug users who have tried to enter a treatment program and been turned away. Minorities are disproportionately overrepresented in the ranks of the city's 200,000 IV drug users, and likely comprise a large percentage of those seeking treatment for drug addiction. But to conclude, as you apparently do, that a study of IV drug user behavior therefore automatically targets minorities because of this overrepresentation is to illogically confuse cause with effect.

Finally, by outlandishly charging that "somebody has a brother in the needle business," and irresponsibly echoing the outrageous assertion that I ought to be arrested for murder, you fan the flames of divisiveness and racial hatred in the context of what is already an emotionally charged debate.

You owe your readers an unflinching and understandable description of the devastating dimensions of AIDS.

I never heard back from Mr. Tatum.

Of the major daily newspapers in the city, the *New York Times* and *Newsday* supported the program, the *Post* was negative, and the

*Daily News* took up an anti-needle exchange stance that became increasingly shrill as the months brought the mayoral primary campaign closer. On Oct. 6, for example, the *News* said:

### HALT NEEDLE MADNESS BEFORE IT KILLS

An insanity is about to be turned loose on the streets of New York unless reasonable men and women unite to smash it. That lunacy is a program to give narcotics addicts free needles and syringes, together with a license to escape prohibition of possession of dope paraphernalia. . . . Mayor Koch expressed prudent skepticism about the idea long ago. He then deferred to Joseph. Koch alone could stop it now. He could—and must —simply order Joseph to desist. Halt. Cease. Others must cry out before it begins—or be held accountable.

*Daily News* columnist Earl Caldwell proclaimed, "Once again, it's blacks against the city."

Shortly before the program was about to begin, the *News* printed an editorial that appeared to be calculated to incite the very disorder that it prophesied:

### IT'S UP TO KOCH TO STOP THE NEEDLES

New York's free needle program is just over the horizon. Health Commissioner Stephen Joseph says it will start early in November. No matter what anyone else wants or thinks. Nothing has deflected Joseph from his passion to start handing out hypodermic needles and syringes. Not even the overwhelming community opposition—especially in the black community . . . to hand out free needles bespeaks the grossest insensitivity to the realities of life in New York. What comes next? That's up to Ed Koch. He still has a week to head Joseph off at the pass by countermanding the free-needle program. If he must replace Joseph in order to kill the program once and for all, so be it. But what if Koch fails to act? Community protest would be both inevitable and understandable. People who live near the pilot needle distribution sites . . . cannot be expected to sit quietly by while addicts waltz or slither in to pick up free needles. And that may be only the beginning. Law enforcement officials are already talking quietly about the moral imperative of combating Joseph's irresponsible, inflammatory plan by arresting the addicts who take part in it. To set the Health Department against the police and prosecutors—local and federal —would be an act of sheer madness. Every responsible citizen in New York is on the same side in the War on Drugs. It is time for Ed Koch to call the ranks to order—by killing the misbegotten free-needle program before it starts.

As the pressure mounted, I knew that this would be the test of my relationship with Ed Koch. There was nothing but political trouble for him in his continued support of "my" program, a program about which his own feelings were positive but skeptical. I had observed that he strongly supported those commissioners in whom he had basic confidence up to the point where they became intolerable liabilities and he chucked them over the side. That was fine with me. I always felt that this way I knew where I stood with the Mayor, and was prepared to stake my job on the merits of my arguments.

Though I was saddened and, to be frank, hurt by the allegations of racism, I felt secure in my assessment of the importance and value of the program. As I said in a letter in response to the *Daily News* editorial attack (a letter that they published on October 31):

Dubiousness, hesitancy, and even heated popular opposition have historically been hallmarks of many crucial public health initiatives, from sanitation to vaccination to fluoridation. But the News's recent attempt to fan the flames of irrationality and whoop up neighborhood hysteria, all in the name of strangling the Health Department's needle-exchange study in the cradle, is inexcusable. . . . As the person charged with protecting the health of this city's people, I must take every reasonable measure available to me to arrest the rampaging AIDS virus. I believe this study reasonable, based on dispassionate review of the evidence before me.

Each day during this period I wondered if I would get a call from First Deputy Mayor Stan Brezenoff or from the Mayor telling me to back off, or offering me the chance to clean out my desk. But that call never came, on this or any other issue. Even when the Mayor disagreed with my position, and on the few occasions when he over-ruled me, he never asked that I restrain my rhetoric, or abandon a professional position of my own to make his political one easier.

As the days drew near the proposed early November start of the program, two events occurred that once again almost did us in. The first was a tragedy: two New York City police officers were shot and killed on the same day in drug-related incidents. The public was furious, and it was only natural, if illogical, to link the needle ex-change to that outrage.

But still the Mayor stood firm. Not only did he not "cut me off at the pass" as the *Daily News* had urged, but he still supported the plan publicly: "I don't know if this experiment will work," he said in response to the Council's Minority Caucus demands that he kill the program, "but I certainly think we have to explore it and test it."

The second event was another in that sequence that almost stopped the program before it began, and it was compounded of symbolism, hysteria, and a severe tactical error on the part of myself and my staff.

The placement of the sites for needle exchange had always been a thorny issue. For the small-scale project of 200 addicts exchanging needles, we had planned to use two test sites and also two control sites (where another 200 addicts would get counseling, drug treat-ment referral, and all the other components of the program except clean needles). We planned to use space within four of our thirteen widely scattered district health centers for these purposes and to choose, of course, centers where there was a specially high preva-lence of drug use in the surrounding community.

We knew, of course, that the exchange sites would provoke a kind of "Super-NIMBY (Not In My Backyard)" response, and that no City Council member or other community leader would entertain the prospect without loud and strong objection. The only way to get the program going was to choose the sites by the best program criteria we could, and then make our argument that we were conducting a Health Department program in an existing Health Department building. There was even a weak precedent; we already had one health center in Manhattan that included a methadone maintenance program within the same building.

As the start of the program drew near, I discussed the problem with Stan Brezenoff and the Mayor; we agreed that the Health Department would select the sites on the merits, and that I would give the City Council representatives concerned advance notice.

The sites chosen for needle exchange included our Chelsea Health Center in lower Manhattan (a predominantly white area) and the Bushwick Health Center in Brooklyn (predominantly Hispanic). The control sites were to be on the Upper West Side of Manhattan at the Riverside Health Center (predominantly Hispanic) and at the Crown Heights Health Center in Brooklyn (predominantly black). All these areas have heavy drug dealing and drug use, and we hoped we could escape the hysteria that the program was "bringing large numbers of addicts from 'outside the community' to endanger our streets."

Our hopes were, of course, to no avail. As soon as the news became public (and it was general knowledge within hours after telling individual council members), a new storm of protest and controversy rose up. No one wanted the program on "their" streets. Everyone had an argument for why, if it had to begin at all, it should begin in someone else's neighborhood.

The Chelsea community, one of the best organized communities in the city, and experienced in this area—it had blocked a methadone program a few years previously—threw the blockbuster: the health center where the needle exchange was to take place was adjacent to a primary school! This fueled community uproar along the general lines that the addicts using the program would endanger or corrupt the children. In vain I tried to point out that the "drug addicts" were the neighbors—sometimes the parents—of the children, that one could pick up scores of crack vials in the streets surrounding the school and health center every morning, and that a significant proportion of the very same patients who visited the sexually transmitted disease, AIDS testing, and tuberculosis clinics daily were the prospective clients of the needle exchange project in the same building. The image of the school next to the drug clinic was too great.

We met with community residents and political leaders, but could not overcome the pressures that had been generated by the revelation that a public elementary school, a parochial school, and several daycare centers were all within several blocks of the health center.

In response to the barrage of criticism, the Mayor announced on television that he would instruct me not to locate any needle exchange sites (including the control sites, where no needles would actually be exchanged) within a thousand feet of any elementary school or daycare center, a prohibition similar to the statute prohibiting liquor sales within a thousand feet of a school.

We had, frankly, just missed the ball. In a dense urban landscape, the fact that a health center was cheek-by-jowl with elementary and nursery schools had not registered with significance. I quickly sent staff out to check the environs of all of our health centers, and the news was, to put it mildly, not good. There was not a single health center in the city that did not have one, or several, schools and daycare centers within a block or two (after all, where do you try to locate health centers, if not near schools?). None of our centers was usable, no non-Health Department site (such as the public hospitals) would accept the program, and it looked as if we were out of business.

But I still believed that this was too important an effort to be stymied, and the Mayor said he would still support the program if we could find an acceptable site.

We circled the wagons, and looked within our own Health Department headquarters, located in lower Manhattan, a nonresidential area in the midst of official city, state, and federal office buildings. The Health Department is located among court buildings, not far from City Hall, the Police Department, and the Criminal Court. Hardly an auspicious environment in which to begin a "user-friendly" needle exchange, but it was, quite literally, all we had.

We identified a small storage area on the ground floor that was stocked with janitorial supplies and old X rays, cleaned it out, spruced it up, filled it with a small program staff whose caring and competence were matched by their irrepressible morale, and announced we would open, as scheduled, on November 7, 1988.

After two and a half years, it had come down to a tiny program in a broom closet, but we were going to make it work.

As we approached Monday, November 7, we had threats of demonstrations by Hilton Clark, who was still shouting genocide, promises of counter-demonstrations by ADAPT supporting the program, threats of lawsuits by the City Council's Minority Caucus, and another salvo from Police Commissioner Ward, who said, "As a black person, we have a particular sensitivity to doctors conducting experiments, and they too frequently seem to be conducted against blacks."

With all the publicity, and the site constraints, we expected a slow start. On Tuesday—after three years of debate and one day of program—the *New York Times* wrote a premature obituary:

> Only two drug addicts showed up yesterday to receive free needles on the first day of New York City's controversial experiment aimed at slowing the spread of AIDS, health officials said. Despite the low turnout, the city Health Commissioner, Stephen C. Joseph, who has championed the needle exchange program in the face of heated criticism from a variety of sources, said he was pleased. "I think the enormous success of today is that the program got off the ground at all," he said. "Nobody stopped us from doing it." . . . Dr. Joseph said his counselors had found a drug rehabilitation program, starting today, for one of the two men who came in yesterday. The other is to start in about a week. "One of the brightest parts of the day," said Dr. Joseph, "is that we have two people set for treatment, and we have given them a safe bridge until they get there."

The program grew slowly but surely. After all the prophecies of disaster and social discord, we did not have a single disruptive client, nor a single police-related episode. Thousands of city employees and members of the public walked through the first floor of the Health Department daily (birth, death, and other vital records are available to the public there); no thefts or assaults took place. No complaints of needles jettisoned in the street near the program were received; no occasions of "Health Department needles" being sold to children or adults were encountered.

The program went so smoothly in large part because of the quality of the program director, Chuck Eaton, and his small staff of counselors. All were experienced drug treatment workers; Chuck himself had left the directorship of one of the city's major methadone treatment programs to come to work for needle exchange because he believed in it. The staff was moved by a commitment to help people get off drugs, and to protect them from AIDS while they were getting there. Ironically, the constraints on the program's size worked to its benefit, giving the counselors adequate time to spend with clients, to gain their trust and confidence, and to search the city by phone looking for an available and appropriate treatment spot for each individual.

Since the ground rules of the program were that only persons who had been refused entry to drug treatment would be enrolled, we were dependent upon the city's existing drug treatment programs for referrals. Our experience here was mixed; some clinics were enthusiastic sources of referral, others were hostile, most were indifferent. Transportation from all over the city to lower Manhattan was a major problem; we provided transport and subway tokens, but the system was cumbersome.

Slowly we grew: 2 clients the first day, 8 at the end of a week, 32 after a month, 74 at 2 months. Opposition persisted: the *Daily News* kept up a drumbeat of criticism, the City Council petitioned the Mayor and Dr. Axelrod to shut us down (both defended the continuation of the program).

Behind the small success, however, was another reality: the program was crippled by its small size and inappropriate location. I was by now sure that we would "prove" that we could survive, and operate on a very restricted scale, but the experiment was, in the larger sense, artificial. Though the program was nationally visible as needle exchange, we were more accurately getting a very small number of addicts into drug treatment, and supporting them briefly with clean needles and education while they waited for a treatment spot to open.

In late February 1989, I petitioned David Axelrod to let us expand the program to include addicts who could come to us straight from the street—not solely via the intermediary of a drug treatment program that had no room for them. Dr. Axelrod was supportive of this direction of expansion. Meantime, we were searching for other sites. I wrote and called voluntary hospitals, drug treatment programs, churches and community service groups, looking for several nongovernment groups who might give us sanctuary from the thousand-foot rule, thinking that if I found the private sites I might talk the Mayor into letting me go ahead, especially since the initial program was working. I had several nibbles but no promises; it was a maddeningly frustrating business, trying to jack up two ends without assurance at the middle.

The staff was constantly challenging me with new proposals to find and attract clients, all of them sound public health recruitment ideas. I would be faced with trying to decide which ones we could get away with, and which might bring down the program around our ears. Should we canvas several homeless men's shelters? Was it legitimate for us to recruit addicts on the street and take them to drug treatment programs which would reject them, and then bring them ourselves to our program? Could we short-cut the rejection process to a telephone call? I pushed as close to the limit as I dared.

By May I had several additional sites loosely lined up. All were in private or voluntary institutions, all were in high drug-use areas. I went to the Mayor, and proposed that we expand the program into nongovernment sites out in the communities.

Somewhat to my surprise he agreed, requiring only that I wait until after the election primary in September before throwing the fat into the fire again. We were ready for expansion to a meaningful community-based program—but it was not to work out that way.

All three other mayoral candidates had declared their opposition to needle exchange, and vowed to kill the program if elected. If the next Mayor was Democrat David Dinkins, Republican Rudolph Giuliani, or Conservative Ronald Lauder, the needle exchange would be dismantled. When David Dinkins defeated Ed Koch in the Democratic primary in early September, we knew the end was near. We continued with our broom-closet program, trying to learn as much as we could, and achieve as much as we could, in the time left to us. In early December, the department prepared a report on the first year entitled *The Pilot Needle Exchange Study in New York City: A Bridge to Treatment*, thus emphasizing the character of the program.

In my transmittal letter to David Axelrod, I emphasized our findings: injection drug users can be motivated to change their behavior in significant health-enhancing ways; coordinated supportive services can be provided compassionately and cost-effectively; the distribution of needles and syringes in conjunction with counseling and health services did not result in community disruption or a significant change in the public perception of the city's overall "anti-drug use" stance.

In sum, no indicators of harm, and several significant indicators of benefits, resulted from our first, and only, year of experience.

The department had recruited 294 persons into needle exchange; over half of them were HIV-antibody positive. More than 75 percent accepted referral to a drug treatment program, and at least half of these have entered treatment; of 56 clients who were confirmed to have entered treatment, more than half were still in treatment 60 days later. These figures, though too fragmentary to give firm conclusions, are comparable to the best results reported from traditional drug treatment programs.

The political realities of New York City seriously flawed the execution of the pilot program; most damaging was the restriction of the program site to a central Department of Health location. The small scale and uncertainties of the activity preclude any rigorous analysis of the program's outcomes. And, of course, the tiny scale of the program, only engaging one out of every thousand intravenous drug users, was much too small to have any impact on the problem of AIDS transmission. After three years of enormous travail, had the elephant given birth to a flea?

Nevertheless, the pilot program demonstrated that needle exchange could be carried out, even in a very hostile environment, that it could not be shown to lead to any harmful effects, and that there were some preliminary indications of benefits. Given the scope and urgency of the AIDS crisis, and the lack of other demonstrable remedies, the clear lesson from the pilot program should have been to expand efforts to a wider scale, and to continue to attempt to measure the effects of needle exchange on both drug and AIDS-related behavior. When one is hanging over a cliff, even a half-inch of progress generally gives a clear idea of how to proceed further.

Shortly after his election as Mayor, David Dinkins made good on his campaign promise to end needle exchange. I had sent him a letter along with our year-end report, urging that he examine the evidence before he acted. No reply was ever received.

The new Commissioner of Health, Dr. Woodrow Meyers, declared himself in fundamental opposition ("on a theological basis," according to the *New York Times*) not only to needle exchange, but also to the distribution of bleach and to the education of drug addicts in the cleaning of injection equipment, and threatened to withhold city funds for those purposes from the 1990 Department of Health contract with ADAPT. By May 1990, several groups in the city were engaged in street distribution of needles and syringes as a measure of civil disobedience.

We had come full circle.

There are two postscripts to this story of needle exchange in New York City. They each concern another of those bizarre twists and turns in the AIDS epidemic that would leave readers skeptical if it were to be written as fiction. But this is, indeed, what happened.

The street needle exchange activity undertaken as civil disobedience after Mayor David Dinkins closed down the Department of Health program was led by members of ACT-UP. The leaders of this campaign were arrested in May of 1990 as they handed out needles and syringes to addicts in lower Manhattan.

The following spring they came to trial; their defense was, as it had been when another group of ACT-UP members had occupied my office in the Department of Health in 1988, a plea of necessity, a need to act because of the exigencies of the AIDS epidemic. Indeed, several members of the group arrested for passing out needles were the same individuals who had been convicted in the prior criminal trespass case.

The ACT-UP defendants asked me to testify as a major witness on their behalf, and I agreed. In my testimony I stated that the closure of the city's official needle exchange program left the defendants no choice but to take the actions that they did, to try and save lives.

The judge hearing the needle exchange case was Laura Drager, the selfsame judge who had rejected the plea of necessity and found the defendants guilty in the prior criminal trespass case in which I was the complainant.

Judge Drager found all the needle exchange defendants innocent —by reason of necessity.

And then, in May 1992, the wheel took one more turn. With a flourish of trumpets, Mayor Dinkins proclaimed that the city would undertake a major needle exchange program, using funds from New York State and the American Foundation for AIDS Research.

The same administration that had joined the chorus in accusing us of the most reprehensible motives, that had killed our first fledgling program in 1990, whose new Health Commissioner had proclaimed needle exchange immoral, and whose lawyers had opposed us in the 1991 trial of the ACT-UP needle exchange defendants, now asserted that they were mounting a major needle exchange effort that would avoid the flaws of small scope of our initial program.

The thousands of men, women, and children whose HIV infections could have been prevented would have been better served if David Dinkins had put his shoulder to the wheel with us when we began the struggle, almost six years to the day earlier.

# 9

## *Drugs, Sex, and AIDS*

We should be talking about abstinence. . . . If we can't make prisoners abstain from illegal and illicit sex, who in the world can we?

> Council Majority Leader Peter Vallone, who also called the distribution of condoms to prison inmates "stupid and mind-boggling."

DESPITE A 1983 STATEMENT IN THE CENTERS FOR DISEASE CONTROL'S weekly reports that, "conceivably, these male drug abusers are carriers of an infectious agent that has not made them ill but caused AIDS in their infected female sexual partners," AIDS in intravenous drug use was for a time considered to be largely a problem of the drug user himself or, more rarely, herself.

The epidemic of drug abuse had festered in the United States for thirty years prior to the arrival of the HIVirus. By the late 1970s, the nation was estimated to have about one million IV drug users, about a quarter of them in New York City. Some 80–90 percent were males and mostly black or Hispanic, in the urban poor neighborhoods where drug sales flourished.

In 1980, the heroin-injecting population had seemed to be aging, with the typical addict in his mid or late thirties, with a long-term habit. There were, however, enough new and younger recruits to keep the population at about the same size as older addicts died off or, less commonly, stopped injecting.

As with many social indicators in public health, especially those associated with illegal or stigmatized behavior, exact information on the numbers and distribution of IV drug users was hard to come by. Should the estimates include only daily users, or also occasional and weekend injectors? Heroin addicts only? What about the increasing numbers of people injecting cocaine, or combining heroin and cocaine in "speedballing"? Should "skin-popping" be included, or only IV injection? Still, the estimates from both law enforcement and public health sources were consistently consonant with the drug-user profile given here.

As the model of an infectious agent, probably a virus, gained credence as the cause of AIDS, it fit very well with patterns of other infections that were prevalent among IV drug injectors. Bloodstream and heart valve bacterial infections were contracted through the sharing of infected injection equipment, the individual use of unsterile needles and syringes, and the puncture of needles through unwashed and contaminated skin. An epidemic of hepatitis B, spread by both blood-to-blood and sexual transmission, had been rampaging for a decade among IV drug users. Hepatitis B, though much more easily communicable from person to person than the HIVirus, became an appropriate model for understanding the transfer of HIV among persons at risk; hepatitis B had also become epidemic among gay males in the 1970s.

The HIVirus had most probably first entered the IV drug using population via infected homosexual men who were also drug injectors. Consistently, 3–4 percent of men with AIDS in New York have had the dual risks of both sex with other men and drug use.

We now know, however, that the initial idea that IV drug users formed a "second wave" of the epidemic, lagging by some years behind the spread of the virus among gay men, was incorrect. Rather, the virus spread very rapidly among IV drug users in the late 1970s, coinciding with the most rapid spread among gay men. Since middle-class gay men were more visible to the health care system than IV drug users, cases of AIDS among gay men were more readily recognized early, but the rising curves of infection in the two populations were roughly parallel.

It is theoretically possible that the virus first entered the drug-injecting population and then spread from them to homosexual men, but the early intense pattern of HIV infection among gay men in cities such as San Francisco and Los Angeles, where rates of HIV infection among IV drug users have remained quite low until recently, make that hypothesis unlikely. It is also possible that the virus entered the two populations independently on several occasions from African or Caribbean sources, and then continued to pass back and forth between them.

We have seen in earlier chapters how the movement of the virus into poor communities was characterized by increasing heterosexual transmission with consequent infection of women and their children, with drug abuse as the engine driving the shift.

Thus, by the middle of the first decade of the epidemic, a very broad and deep band of HIV infection was present among IV drug users, their female sex partners, and their newborn children. This band of infection was, and remains, concentrated in poor neighborhoods and among minority residents, with increasing heterosexual transmission of the virus within these neighborhoods.

In addition to the difficulty of reaching the drug users with prevention education, and the doubled difficulties of reaching addicts and their sexual partners with safer sex messages, was this difficulty: the scarcity of drug treatment, which can prevent the infected addict from continuing to infect others.

The history of treating IV drug addiction has been characterized more by failure and inadequacy than by success. Neither the physiology nor the sociology of addiction is understood well enough to generate confidence about treatment. Basic disagreements abound as to the extent that addiction is a medical or a social phenomenon.

The two major models of heroin treatment are drug-free and methadone maintenance. Drug-free treatment, most often involving twelve to eighteen months of residential care, is expensive (about $15,000 per person per year in public sector programs), intensive in time and resources and, in New York State, accounts for less than a quarter of the 40,000 available treatment spaces. Experts disagree about the true success rates, particularly for patients who lack strong social support to help them through the difficult times during and after treatment. The dropout and relapse rates are very high, exceeding 50 percent in most surveys.

A chemical analogue to morphine and heroin having a similar

addictive potential but far less euphoria than heroin, methadone has been used as a specific chemical means of treating heroin addiction since the mid-1960s. It is, in essence, a substitutive therapy, on which a patient can be maintained indefinitely, or from which some patients can be progressively weaned to abstinence.

Methadone treatment is relatively inexpensive—generally between a fifth and a tenth of the cost of residential drug-free treatment—and is provided on an ambulatory basis (sometimes after brief hospitalization or residential treatment). It has been highly criticized, especially by black community leaders, as a "substitute addiction" that evades the actual problem. Methadone's success is as hard to quantify as drug-free treatment, but not noticeably superior. Taken orally rather than injected, methadone can be "diverted" by patients and sold on the street—and thus can be used by the addict to diminish heroin requirements while continuing drug abuse, such as cocaine, against which methadone is not effective.

Methadone's proponents point out that maintenance programs have enabled thousands of people to lead productive family lives, hold jobs, and avoid the criminal behavior necessary to sustain an expensive and illegal heroin addiction. Methadone's detractors denounce it as continued chemical enslavement sanctioned by a society that does not really care about preventing, curing, or rehabilitating addiction.

Neither drug treatment has been able to affect significantly the numbers of heroin addicts in New York or nationally, but advocates of increased treatment stress that many thousands of individuals have been helped to recovery.

Treatment is relatively scarce. With over 200,000 IV drug users and only 40,000–45,000 drug treatment slots, the city is clearly offering inadequate treatment. Worse, the waiting period for entry to methadone maintenance ranges up to three months, for drug-free treatment up to six months. And while there is almost daily turnover in individual programs, an available opening may be far from the neighborhood of the addict seeking entry into treatment. Yet no new treatment facilities have been opened in New York City in the past fifteen years, in large part because of community resistance.

Even if communities were willing to take the facilities, funds to create and operate them are scarce. Most treatment programs are overseen by a state agency funded with 60 percent federal funds and 40 percent state. Current estimates, which are highly speculative, are that offering treatment to all addicts who would use it, would cost somewhere up to $1 billion annually for New York City alone.

In New York City, as everywhere in the United States, drug abuse prevention and anti-drug law enforcement efforts are far short of the quantity and quality it would take to have a major impact on the drug epidemic, if indeed we were serious about doing so. In New York City and elsewhere, there has been no reduction in the availability of drugs; the street prices of heroin and cocaine have actually decreased since 1980.

By late 1986 or early 1987, awareness was dawning in New York, New Jersey, and elsewhere about the vast scope of HIV infection among IV drug users, and the direct implications that this has for heterosexual transmission and wider infection, especially among minority women. Because of the lack of widespread HIV antibody testing, much of the early evidence was indirect, but it was increasingly persuasive, especially with regard to the rise in other infections that were presumed to reflect widespread immune deficiency from HIV infection. In parts of the South Bronx, rates of pneumonia hospitalization among young women climbed five to tenfold over several years. Tuberculosis rates citywide increased 50 percent over eight years, mostly in young adult black and Hispanic males. Most persuasively, deaths from a variety of infections among IV drug addicts rose sharply between 1980 and 1985, while deaths from drug overdoses remained relatively constant. For example, 92 addicts died of bacterial infections of the heart valves in 1985; the number of such deaths had been only 39 in 1980; 252 addicts died of nonspecific pneumonias in 1985, compared with only 39 in 1980.

The most likely explanation was the spread of silent HIV infection among IV drug users and their sexual partners, leaving large numbers of undiagnosed individuals with early immune deficiency, clinically unrecognized but predisposing them to other infections. Health Department epidemiologists estimated that the actual prevalence of HIV-related illness and deaths that had occurred among IV

drug users was half-again greater than the number of formally diagnosed cases of AIDS in this group.

Dr. Rand Stoneburner and his colleagues at the Department of
Health went back through the medical records of all drug-related
deaths in the city between 1980 and 1986, and found an additional
2,500 deaths that seemed to be HIV-related, but which did not meet
the federal definition of AIDS and had not been so diagnosed. If the
city's mortality figures had been readjusted to take account of these
findings, AIDS-related deaths among IV drug users would have surpassed those among gay men during the early phase of the epidemic, reversing the previous ratio in which AIDS deaths among
gay men accounted for more than 50 percent of the total.

From the recognition of the importance of this channel of HIV
infection, four critical perspectives emerged in 1987–88. First, the
Department of Health recognized that IV drug abuse had been the
main route of HIV infection among addicts, women, and children:
80 percent of the first 1,500 cases of AIDS in women had been IV
drug users or the sex partners of IV drug users. Almost 90 percent of
children with AIDS were the offspring of a drug-injecting parent or
parents. HIV infection in heterosexuals was primarily linked to drug
use. The development of a large existing pool of infected individuals
as the virus spread among drug injectors in minority communities
provided the base from which secondary spread among heterosexual
partners could, and did, take place.

Second, the department saw that spread of HIV infection was
increasing rapidly in poor and minority communities. The women at
highest risk in the newborn antibody testing studies were black and
Hispanic; 60 percent were on Medicaid.

Third, the epidemic was increasing as well as broadening. By
entering the minority heterosexual population, the virus opened a
large, diverse, and not readily identifiable new population to risk.
Our increasing awareness of rising numbers of AIDS cases was only
the overlay of a much larger number of asymptomatic (and unidentified) HIV-infected men and women. This began to be frighteningly
apparent by the late 1980s in such studies as one in the emergency
room of a "sentinel hospital" in an area of the Bronx hardest hit by
both AIDS and drugs; men coming to the emergency room for

whatever medical or surgical complaints showed a silent HIV-infection rate of 27 percent!

Finally, the perspective emerged that making any significant inroads in the widening epidemic of HIV infection would require coping with the primary epidemic, the epidemic of substance abuse. As a society, we were then and still are ill-prepared to do this.

The Department of Health did not have the power to increase drug treatment. But I offered the state the scarcest commodity of all in New York City: space. And not just any space, but space that was not subject to community veto.

I proposed that we use space in several of the thirteen Health Department district health centers scattered around the city, making clinic facilities available in evening and pre-9:00 A.M. hours for state-funded drug treatment, probably mostly methadone maintenance. The state Health Department and Division of Substance Abuse Services expressed interest, and I still believe they gave us a verbal commitment in 1988 to fund 1,500 new treatment slots, but the funds never materialized during the more than two years we wrangled with them over the proposal.

Mayor Koch adamantly maintained his long-standing policy of not funding drug treatment with city revenues—of holding to the agreement that had been struck with New York State in 1979 when the city's fiscal crisis had prompted the state to take over funding responsibility for several major programs, including drug treatment. So I was caught in a double bind, with city and state each pointing at the other as the responsible party. In the final months of his mayoralty, in late 1989, Ed Koch agreed to share responsibility with the state to fund a new initiative for expanded drug treatment. Once again we offered the use of health center space, but once again nothing materialized, and the new Dinkins Administration still has the initiative on hold.

Even the initial rumors that we were considering starting drug treatment in the health centers led to community complaints and protests by City Council members in the familiar litany of "not in my backyard, or on my block, or in my district." In actuality, the health centers would have been excellent sites for drug treatment, because they would have let us link substance abuse treatment with other health services, and avoid the usual isolation and fragmentation of drug treatment from other health services that addicts need.

Our critics, though, didn't care whether the centers would work according to health services criteria; they worried about whether the centers would be well-managed—or would be dirty, disruptive, and dangerous, messing up the neighborhood with large numbers of criminal addicts. In any event, we failed in all our efforts to mount additional drug treatment services.

Even a substantial expansion of drug treatment, however, would have made only a minimal public health impact on the epidemic. The iron law of the numbers was frightful: 200,000 IV drug users, of whom at least 100,000 were already infected. Existing treatment accommodated only 40,000 or so. Even if the city could triple drug treatment over the next few years (a most unlikely and herculean accomplishment), and even if 120,000 addicts would then remain in treatment (also unlikely—best estimates were that if treatment were available on demand, up to 70,000 addicts might take advantage of it), the city would still have almost 100,000 untreated IV drug users, at least half of them already infected with HIV. They would stay outside treatment and be a threat of infection to others, both sexually and by shared injection equipment. It was the inexorable pressure and irrefutable logic of this argument that led me to propose, in 1986, the controversial needle exchange program described in the previous chapter.

Expanded drug treatment is a necessary part of an AIDS strategy, but an element resisted at all levels of society. And even if pursued aggressively, it could not by itself begin to cope with the problem in New York.

Other traditional public health measures of disease control, such as widespread antibody testing for infection, mandatory confidential public health reporting of HIV seropositivity, and vigorous contact tracing to warn unsuspecting partners and identify new seropositives were also strongly resisted, especially by gay advocates.

We were left, then, with education and advocacy efforts, which were particularly difficult to implement effectively with IV drug users. We attempted to use all the channels we could think of: mass media campaigns, street outreach workers, funding of community-based groups and institutions working with drug abusers, brochures and pamphlets, support of drug use prevention education, etc. Our messages focused on drug avoidance and the use of clean injection equipment: "Don't shoot up, but if you do, don't share needles. Use clean works, and here is how to clean them." The dual message, as might be expected, led to criticism from religious and other groups that we were "promoting drug use," analogous to criticism of our safer sex education (which also was an important part of our messages to drug users). These charges were a very mild forerunner to the criticism we were to experience in distributing clean needles and syringes to addicts.

As we were developing our initial proposal for needle exchange, I learned of a program in Los Angeles that was distributing small vials of household bleach to addicts as a measure to clean injection equipment. On September 5, 1986, I sent a memo to staff asking for a fully detailed proposal for a large-scale pilot program to test the effectiveness of distributing small vials of bleach solution to individual addicts and in the galleries—hitting as wide a distribution as possible. I wanted to have this operating by the first week in October, along with a method for evaluating actual usage and effectiveness—nothing elaborate. I also wanted it tied to our distribution of "Clean Works" brochures, carrying the clear connotation "Don't Shoot Up, But if You Must" etc.

Staff response was less than enthusiastic. The consensus was that direct distribution by the department of bleach in New York City would draw as much hostile rhetorical fire as would our proposed needle exchange project, and would carry major liabilities, such as the risk of small children finding the vials and ingesting the bleach. Opposition to bleach distribution might also jeopardize the needle exchange, which we all felt was more important.

I let myself be persuaded to drop the direct distribution of bleach and, as an alternative, to fund a private organization that worked with drug abusers to "do it for us," distributing kits that included condoms, safer sex information, "clean works" instructions, and vials of bleach. In retrospect, I believe that I made a significant error with that decision; the criticism of our needle exchange was so vehement, and the scale of the program we were able to mount so restricted, that we should have taken the added opposition and criticism to gain the added help that a citywide bleach distribution would have offered. I know the Mayor would have supported us. It would have meant another bitter fight, but I think we could have won it. When the needle exchange program was later dismantled as one of the first acts of newly elected Mayor David Dinkins, it would have left the Health Department with at least one strong arrow (bleach distribution) in its quiver.

The city's jail system offered an especially important venue for prevention activities aimed at IV drug users. Some 110,000 individuals come through the city correctional system annually, none sentenced to more than a year, and many revolving through in only a matter of days; the average stay is two weeks. Studies had shown that 50 percent of inmates were current or former IV drug users, and we would expect at least half of them to be infected. That meant a population of 25,000 HIV-infected prisoners a year, with the entire 110,000 important to reach with prevention activities. Since the Department of Health provided health services in the jails, we were well-placed to mount an AIDS prevention and care program, and in this we had open and full cooperation from Correction Commissioner Richard J. Koehler.

Our Prison Health Services began by trying to improve clinical services for prisoners diagnosed with AIDS and housed in individual cells in the prison infirmary on Rikers Island. This did not permit adequate nursing or medical care. We worked with the Department of Correction to design and construct a separate dormitory building for prisoners with diagnosed HIV disease who were not ill enough to be hospitalized in Bellevue or other city hospitals. Once a prisoner was diagnosed with HIV disease, he was placed in this unit and not returned to the general jail population. The many other HIV-positive prisoners were not segregated, nor were they forcibly tested. However, from both the Correction and Health points of view, a prisoner known to have AIDS was safer by far in the separate unit, which by 1989 was housing sixty inmates, with construction underway to double that capacity. By 1988, over half of the roughly forty deaths among New York City prisoners each year were due to HIV illness. There were enormous complexities in providing medical confidentiality and adequate treatment to this group, whose clinical conditions changed rapidly from acute illness requiring hospitalization to ambulatory status and back again.

We mounted a broad-based program of education for inmates and their visitors detailing risk avoidance concerning sex and drug practices that transmit HIV, along with a discharge pack of educational materials and condoms upon release from jail. We also provided AIDS education to Correction staff to diminish anxiety and increase a realistic understanding of risk and prevention. In a joint effort among the Departments of Health and Correction, the Health and Hospitals Corporation (which runs the municipal hospitals), and the district attorneys, we worked out and implemented by 1987 a program of expanded compassionate release for those prisoners dying of AIDS who could be released to die at home.

The prevalence of the HIVirus among jail inmates made the availability of condoms crucial for those who might engage in consensual sex while in jail. This proposal, of course, drew the ire of the moralists. It seemed inadmissible to acknowledge that consensual homosexual sex took place in the city jails, though every authority knew this to be a fact of prison life. Many Correction officials also were more logically opposed to condoms in the prisons because of their use in drug smuggling (the drugs swallowed inside a tied-off condom, and then retrieved later from feces).

The same old tired cry was heard again: you are condoning and promoting immorality. And our response was the same: we are trying to save lives and prevent further infection in an epidemic.

To win this battle, we developed a simple but effective secret weapon: a study of all inmates diagnosed by the Prison Health Services with gonorrhea, whether anal, oral, or urethral, over a three-month period. The incubation period of gonorrhea is two to seven days, ten at most. Thus those who first develop symptoms ten days or more after incarceration must have been infected while in jail. The study showed that at least 10–15 percent of men diagnosed with gonorrhea must have been infected after they were incarcerated, and thus must have engaged in sexual activity while in jail. This made it hard to argue with a proposal that would provide condoms, under medical auspices, to those at high risk.

The Mayor backed my proposal, in part because Correction Commissioner Koehler had the courage to go against the conventional wisdom of his field. We worked out a program by which sexual activity was still officially forbidden in the jails, and condoms were still banned, but "Health Department condoms" would be deliberately overlooked by guards during cell searches and prescribed to prisoners who requested them, initially to men who had asked to be housed in a separate facility for homosexuals, then to a wider prison population. The furor died down; we prescribed our condoms. I do not know precisely how much HIV transmission we prevented in the jails, but certainly some.

We also began a program of voluntary HIV antibody testing in the jails, within a system of closely guarded medical confidentiality of test results, which were not shared with Correction staff. Of the first 500 prisoners who asked to be tested, over half were positive!

Coping with AIDS in prison will remain enormously complex, combining a thicket of challenges to adequate clinical care, safeguarding the rights of infected (and uninfected) prisoners, and avoiding penal and judicial abuse of HIV-infected prisoners. Nowhere do the channels of sex, drugs, and AIDS come closer together than in prison, which presents difficult challenges but also unparalleled opportunities for prevention.

Just as we began to think in 1987 and 1988 that we had grasped the essence of the drugs and AIDS interaction via heroin, the epidemic took another one of those unexpected turns it has a special predilection for. The rules of drugs, sex, and AIDS changed again and, as no one had envisaged, cocaine became the engine driving the future of the AIDS epidemic. Crack—a highly purified, smokable form of cocaine—entered the New York City drug scene in late 1984; most health workers had never heard of it until 1986.

Crack represented a brilliant marketing strategy on the part of drug dealers and suppliers. A widely desired illegal substance that produced feelings of euphoria and power, cocaine had been given great chic through its quasi-legitimatization by athletes and media stars, and its near open use by fashionable people in the 1970s and 1980s. It sold on the streets for about $50 per unit of purchase. Some sophisticated users "free-based," that is, they purified the cocaine by heating it with ether or other solvents (a very dangerous practice, due to the explosive potential of the solvents heated over a stove or an open flame), and then inhaled the purified product for an accentuated and accelerated rush through direct absorption in the lungs.

The advantages of crack to the drug dealers were stupendous. Here was cocaine packaged in a form that could be sold at $5 or $10, one-tenth the unit price, and which could be taken without the risk or mess of IV heroin or cocaine injection. Crack gave a much faster and more intense high and a steeper and deeper down, thus accelerating the desire for repeat administration, binge use, and true addiction.

Crack is highly purified cocaine (cocaine is usually sold at 10–25 percent purity on the street), brought to about 90 percent purity by heating with another compound, usually sodium bicarbonate. The process can be undertaken safely on a kitchen stove, with materials readily obtainable. Crack, as opposed to free-based cocaine, appears in the form of nonexplosive crystals which are smoked by heating them in a small glass or plastic pipe. The result is delivered straight to the rich absorptive vascular bed in the lungs, and thus to the brain, accelerating the time of onset of action of the drug to several seconds rather than the several minutes required for snorted cocaine.

The name "crack" is said to have several origins. Some say it is because the coke is "cracked" by heating; some say the small crystals look like the cracked plaster in deteriorated housing; some say the name comes from the crackling sound it makes in the pipe. In some parts of the country, it is called "rock," another allusion to its crystalline form.

Whatever the derivation of its name, it is cheap to make, easy to sell, and leads to a flood of entrepreneurship in the drug trade. A rash of adolescent street dealers as young as thirteen carrying telephone beepers, and preteens who act as lookouts and runners, can produce and sell crack as middlemen. Because crack involves no injection and because it can be sold so cheaply, it addicts ever younger children. And the proportion of women among crack addicts is far higher than among heroin injectors.

If your intention were to develop a large and insatiable market for drug abuse, crack would be as close to an ideal product as you could imagine.

Crack hit New York City like a blizzard in the mid-1980s. Law enforcement agencies were helpless to control its distribution or use. By 1987 it was sold openly on many streets. The city had fewer than 10,000 drug treatment spaces that could be used for crack addicts. In any event, no proven effective measure for treating cocaine addiction existed, even if the city had had space in treatment facilities, which were already full to bursting with heroin addicts. There was, quite simply, no place for crack addicts to go for treatment, even when they wanted to. The city had no reliable estimates of the numbers of heavy crack users, but a safe guess is around 200,000.

Crack's arrival was catastrophic. The violent and paranoid behavior associated with its addiction led to steep increases in assault and murder. The domination of the street-supply market by violent adolescents and young adult males with easy access to illegal automatic weapons drove up the homicide rate—1990 showed more than a 20 percent increase over 1989. Street gangs warring for control of drug-dealing territory—using Uzis rather than the knives and bats of more innocent days—accounted for a steady stream of casualties, many of them innocent bystanders (including infants and small children) shot by accident in the line of fire, or as random targets to prove a murderer's bona fides.

In addition, the city endured another crisis in child abuse and neglect. Reported cases of child abuse went from 18,000 in 1980 to 55,000 in 1988. The foster care caseload, which had fallen from 20,000 in 1980 to about 16,000 in 1984, jumped back to 24,000 in 1988. Not all of the increase was drug-related of course, but much was. In 1985, for example, 1,325 infant foster care cases were drug-related; only two years later, the number had almost quadrupled to 4,263.

The Health Department tracks maternal drug abuse on birth certificates, a useful public health measure, though one which gives an underestimate of drug abuse and addiction. Between 1980 and 1988, the prevalence of maternal cocaine abuse increased twentyfold, accounting for more than 70 percent of recorded maternal drug abuse. Almost all of this was crack use, nonexistent before 1985. The profile of cocaine users derived from birth certificates showed maternal abusers who were seven times more likely than nonabusers to have had late or no prenatal care; more than twice as likely to be black and to lack health insurance; more than four times as likely to have a sexually transmitted disease.

Infants of cocaine abusers were four times as likely to be of low birth weight, and over a third of them were premature.

Infants of cocaine-abusing mothers had an infant mortality rate three times the city average, whether the infants were of low birth weight or not.

The crack epidemic intersected exactly in both time and space with the spread of the HIV epidemic into the heterosexual minority communities in New York City. It quickly became the new driving force behind the further propagation of the AIDS epidemic and, as with almost everything else about the epidemic, it had begun to do this before we even knew it was there. The dragon was once more within the gates.

Hypersexual behavior is often associated with heavy cocaine use, and this was also associated with crack, providing increased possibilities for heterosexual HIV transmission among unsuspecting partners. Sex-for-drugs transactions mushroomed in New York, a sort of amateur prostitution by which women financed their crack addiction.

In many neighborhoods, crack activities were centered in crack houses, where crack was produced, sold, and consumed. These crack houses were also centers of sexual activity, often involving young women who, having exhausted their own financial resources, remained in the crack house for hours or days, exchanging sex with other crack house clients for repeated "hits" of the drug. These women, called "strawberries," had sex with men who were often current or former IV drug users; the extreme potential for HIV transmission is obvious.

The crack houses became the next version of the shooting galleries and the gay bathhouses of the early epidemic: unprotected, high-risk behavior with large numbers of often anonymous partners.

The locations of crack houses are often an open secret in their neighborhood. I briefly considered the possibility of sending Health Department staff to the houses to educate and distribute condoms— the department has a tradition of doing this type of work in brothels, for prevention and diagnosis of sexually transmitted diseases, with no publicity and no police involvement. Given the extraordinary hazards and violence of the crack houses, a moment's reflection showed that we could not send staff in. Our street outreach workers did try to concentrate their efforts in heavy crack areas; this was hazardous enough.

With the sexual excesses of the crack epidemic, rates of sexually transmitted diseases skyrocketed. New cases of adult syphilis doubled between 1987 and 1988; for the first time the new cases in women exceeded those reported in men. A year later, the increase was reflected in a doubling of reported congenital syphilis in newborn infants.

Increasingly, crack addicts have turned to injecting cocaine, or combining injectable cocaine and heroin to moderate the cocaine rush. They inject more frequently than do traditional heroin addicts and are more likely to share needles. They are also accelerating the pathway of AIDS transmission via shared needle use.

In addition to its direct effects upon the propagation of the AIDS epidemic, the crack epidemic has also had a series of important indirect effects. At a time when city social and health services have been straining to cope adequately with the burdens of the AIDS epidemic, crack has added to the service needs in all the ways described above. Picture New York's neonatal intensive care hospital units, currently running at 200 percent of capacity, or the stresses produced by boarder babies: these are created even in greater part by the crack epidemic than by cases of pediatric AIDS, although the two are so closely related that they cannot be disentangled.

Since neither the crack epidemic nor the spread of AIDS in minority neighborhoods show any sign of abating, the words of Dr. Margaret Heagarty, Chief of Pediatrics at Harlem Hospital, have more accuracy than poetic license: "We are losing a generation."

In an early attempt at AIDS education for drug users, the Department of Health sponsored a poster contest among current and former drug addicts. My favorite among the winners carries what is probably the most graphic AIDS message ever produced. It shows a needle and syringe. Inside the syringe, blood forms the silhouette of a man and woman embracing. From the tip of the needle emanates a drop of blood in the form of an amniotic sac which contains a fetus. The legend says, "AIDS, Sex, and Drugs: Don't Pass It On."

But of course we have passed it on, without remission, and have not yet found the knowledge, the wisdom, or the social courage to take the steps in law enforcement, education, drug treatment, and public health measures to begin to bring the flow of blood and treasure even partially under control.

## Dealing with Drugs

Any strategy to contain the spread of AIDS must confront ways to ameliorate the abuse of drugs.

The similarities between the epidemics of AIDS and drugs are significant: both are spread through intimate, socially disapproved and, in some cases, illegal behavior. In neither is enough known about the underlying psychosocial determinants, the detailed biological chains of cause and effect, or the effective mechanisms for primary prevention and definitive treatment.

Both epidemics strike particularly at the young: young adults and, increasingly, adolescents. Both find their most explosive expression among population groups who are disadvantaged, discriminated against, and viewed as minorities in one sense or the other.

Both epidemics fit a basic infectious disease transmission model; the drug user is the chief means of recruiting and selling to potential drug users. One infected/addicted person forms a lifelong reservoir of potential infection/addiction of others.

But there is at least one critical difference between the AIDS and drug epidemics. AIDS is caused by a virus; it is not willed, nor does anyone profit; it is then transmitted by largely volitional human behavior, which is what gives some hope of prevention through education and conscious risk reduction.

Drug abuse is also a human behavior—volitional or not, depending on your definition of addiction. But, in contrast to AIDS, a primary cause of the drug epidemic is the deliberate, profit-seeking, conscious sale of illegal substances.

Now suppose, just for a moment, that the paranoid theories about AIDS being a deliberate invention of "biological warfare" were true, which they are not. And suppose that identifiable groups of entrepreneurs were importing and distributing the HIVirus for financial gain (say, to stimulate sales of a miraculous and expensive cure). What do you imagine the societal response would be?

With drugs, there is a clear and definable enemy, which poses a clear and present danger to the nation: those who produce and sell illegal drugs. We have met this clear and present danger with evasion, corruption, knowingly inadequate response, and shallow political cliches (War on Drugs; Just Say No; Drug Czar).

Upon those occasions when society has roused itself to some sort of action, some have believed that the problem might be solved in a short time, with the magic bullet of the moment. On other occasions, society has concluded that the situation is not so desperate, that "recreational" drug use is a universal and perhaps healthy human phenomenon, that it is chic for the beautiful people to snort cocaine, that "alcohol and cigarettes are just as bad, and we don't outlaw those, do we," that "prohibition proved that criminalizing drugs can't work."

What is needed is not the legalization of drugs, but the effective criminalization of the supply, with harsh, swift, and credible sanctions in both foreign and domestic markets. On the demand side, the strategy needs to be equally intensive but quite different: an educational, public health, and medical model that is supportive and therapeutic.

The further spread of the HIVirus will not be stemmed without effective control of the substance abuse epidemic. But even a solution to AIDS that left the drug epidemic intact would be a hollow victory, especially for poor and minority communities that increasingly are to bear the burdens of both epidemics.

An appropriate strategy for overcoming the epidemic of substance abuse, and especially its current and future links with AIDS, would interdict the flow of current drugs of choice as well as forthcoming new drugs, of which crack is the harbinger.

While it would be comforting to think that heroin injection is fading and will collapse of its own weight as the current generation of addicts die off and education regarding the dangers of unsterile injection and needle-sharing take hold, that is likely to prove a delusion. There is no evidence to date of significant success of anti-injection education among addicts. What evidence there is, largely from San Francisco and New York, indicates new patterns of needle use, with injection of cocaine or cocaine-heroin combinations. As the archetypal models of contemporary drug addiction, strong sanctions need to be maintained against the importation, distribution, and possession of heroin and cocaine.

Crack offers many marketing advantages, including the ease of administration without the "mess" and obvious dangers of IV injection. This, combined with its very rapid and intense effects, has made it particularly seductive for adolescents and women. Even as understanding of crack's virulent destructiveness grows, there seems to be little evidence of significant decrease in its use, especially by inner-city young adults.

It is virtually certain that drug suppliers will follow up their brilliant success with crack by developing and marketing other purified smokable derivatives to a population already conditioned by the addiction of cigarette smoking. The most "desirable" characteristics of these new drugs would also follow the crack model: intense euphoria and feelings of powerfulness, heightened sexual expectation, and severe addiction potential.

We are already seeing this pattern in the emergence, particularly in Hawaii and on the West Coast, of "ice" (smokable amphetamine). Obviously, especially given the likelihood that these new drugs will be synthetic or semisynthetic substances, easily produced in large quantities in simple local or even home-based laboratories, the key to any interdiction strategy must rest on seizure at the local, or street level.

There has been widespread debate over the feasibility and desirability of international interdiction of drugs. My own belief is that this is a necessity, for both substantive (in the case of heroin and cocaine) and symbolic reasons. A wide range of diplomatic and military options should be employed, ranging from the withholding of credits and financial assistance from governments that actively or passively participate in production and export of heroin and cocaine to the United States, to development assistance that encourages crop substitution among the local producers and also to direct technical and military assistance to governments in combating drug production in or distribution from their countries.

Covert or overt military involvement of U.S. forces will prove a necessity. Those who are appalled by this statement should weigh this in the context of our willingness to employ military force to protect petroleum products. The longer-term implications of the drug epidemic are at least equally dangerous to the nation's stability and security—the addiction, and therefore destruction, of a large proportion of the country's children.

The most vital focal point of interdiction is at the local level, both transshipments of large quantities of drugs between and within communities, and sales of smaller quantities on the street. This is, of course, especially true for domestically produced and synthetic drugs.

Local interdiction requires serious law enforcement: vastly expanded police presence on the streets, with a primary emphasis on reducing drug sales and drug-related crime; streamlined and expanded court processing for drug-related offenses, with large increases in prison facilities; mandatory sentences for drug-dealing convictions; mandatory drug treatment as an adjunct (not a substitution) to incarceration; and the wide availability of boot-camp "shock incarceration" facilities for convicted prisoners who are drug addicted, but not themselves convicted drug dealers. A concerted effort should be made to provide, either state by state or through a

constitutional amendment, for either life imprisonment without pa-
role or for the death penalty for capital crimes committed in conjunction with drug dealing, and for persons convicted of sale or
distribution of very large quantities of drugs.

As harsh as these measures sound, they are the only ways to
produce an effective deterrent at the street level, especially in larger
cities. Most importantly, they are the only ways to provide a credible buffer so that the efforts of longer-term importance, preventive
education and drug treatment, can have any chance at all to catch
hold on a wide enough scale.

On the user side, we must first realize that we are profoundly
ignorant of the dynamics of addiction, beginning with why people
use drugs in the first place. Abstruse theories abound, but have
been of very little value in translating into drug abuse prevention or
treatment. Knowledge of the biology of addiction is rudimentary.
Several decades of federally funded research has produced prevention and treatment that are flabby at best.

And yet we cannot afford to wait until we have more perfect
knowledge. In combating drug abuse, as with AIDS, we cannot let
the best be the enemy of the good. The only sensible course is to
couple research and action, with constant reinforcement between
one and the other.

Had the same type of aggressively funded and publicly visible
research program been in place on drug addiction as has been put
in place in a few short years regarding AIDS, we would have been
much further ahead on both counts.

Though it is unlikely that any magic bullet will be found either
with regard to addiction in general or (somewhat more likely) with
respect to specific drugs, a hard-driven and coordinated research
program would produce substantial pharmacologic approaches to
substance abuse treatment, and a deeper understanding of the soci-
obiology of addiction would open up new and more effective ave-
nues of prevention and education.

In the meantime, and closely coupled to ongoing research, we
need to expand the use of the tools we have, no matter how blunt
they are. Drug prevention education should begin with the very
first preschool experience, and progress in appropriate technical de-

tail and context right through secondary school. Federal funding in education to the states should be conditioned upon an acceptable drug education plan and its effective implementation from the individual state. The private and voluntary sectors should provide a persistent stream of resources for anti-drug use messages in the mass media.

In any widespread effort at anti-addiction education, tobacco should be squarely included. Substance abuse messages to children would be considerably enhanced by giving up our hypocrisy concerning tobacco use and advertising, a hypocrisy that children and adolescents see easily through.

The question of alcohol is more difficult. Without doubt the addiction potential and the ill effects on health from alcohol, as with tobacco, are even greater than those of heroin or cocaine. However, the moderate social use of alcohol is so generally accepted, and the disbelief of any ill effects from moderate use so pervasive, that I am skeptical of any success for education campaigns that attempt to equate alcohol with heroin or cocaine. Pragmatism would urge capitalizing on the strong social trends against tobacco, but not risking credibility by an emphasis on alcohol as an addictive substance, when used in moderation. Current research pointing to genetic and other biological markers that can identify those with a heightened potential for alcohol addiction may provide a more acceptable basis for convincing society as a whole of the addictiveness of alcohol. Similarly, research into the biological basis of addiction in general might provide the most valuable insights into new methods of both psychosocial and pharmacologic treatment of substance abuse.

Marijuana likewise poses a dilemma. Despite strong arguments that marijuana should be separated from other more socially and physiologically harmful drugs, and legalized, there are at least three overriding arguments to the contrary.

First, newer varieties of marketed marijuana (mostly produced within the United States), have a much higher concentration of the active ingredient than former varieties, and it is by no means clear that they do not pose a significant health risk. Second, the argument that marijuana is a "gateway" drug, especially for adolescents, increasing the likelihood of progression to more dangerous substance use, has not been refuted, and makes much intuitive sense. Finally, if marijuana were to be legalized, the current manufacturers of tobacco products would almost certainly rush into the market. With their manufacturing power and marketing expertise, they would vastly increase marijuana use over a short period of time, particularly among women, youth, and minorities (the most recent successful targets of their tobacco-marketing campaigns). What a terrible message this would be to send out: a virtual call for enlistments on the wrong side in any "War on Drugs"! For the foreseeable future, marijuana should continue to be a substance whose sale, possession, and use are illegal.

The major objective of substance abuse treatment should be to expand the availability of facilities at the community level, so that the clear message is a dual one of a credible deterrent to supply and a ready accessibility of treatment. All methods of treatment, both methadone maintenance and drug-free programs, need expansion, but the escalating future of drugs other than heroin argue for the heaviest emphasis on drug-free programs. Unfortunately, these are also the most expensive, and least certain approaches.

To date, substance abuse treatment has been largely isolated from other primary health care services. The linkage of the AIDS and drug epidemics shows what a fallacy this is: drug treatment must be widely available within major hospitals and health care settings. Federal and state incentives and authority should be employed to create the integration of substance abuse and other health services.

An ambitious program combining both supply and demand sides would be very expensive—some $15 billion per year over the next ten years. Even more daunting, this would not likely be a program showing rapid results, and would need at least a decade to have major impact.

The alternative approach—various proposals for legalization of addictive drugs—ignores several key points. First, any scheme to legalize the sale and use of some drugs to some individuals would have boundaries that the drug entrepreneurs would exploit: sales to minors, in prohibited quantities, new and ever more biologically harmful agents. Second, the proponents of legalization ignore the destructive effects of drugs such as cocaine on individuals and communities. The violent, paranoid behavior associated with cocaine, PCP, and amphetamines would not be lessened by legalizing sales and use. In the short run, in cities such as New York, where hundreds of thousands of children and adolescents live awash in a drug culture, the removal of those feeble barriers that currently exist to drug use would literally push large numbers of young people over the cliff. Finally, we have now seen the massive increase of associated infectious disease with drug abuse: resurgence of sexually transmitted diseases, tuberculosis, hepatitis, and of course, the future of the AIDS epidemic. To legalize addictive drugs would be to inoculate ourselves with these additional plagues.

The seemingly unsolvable problems of crime and social disorganization driven by substance abuse should not stampede us into a posture of surrender and legalization. Far better, though perhaps more difficult, to face up to the needs of dealing with both the supply and demand sides of the epidemic, and to persevere for the decade or more it will take, and the enormous resource expenditures it will entail.

· · ·

The first decade of the AIDS epidemic has been marked by extremes. There has been brilliant research success, heroism, and innovation by AIDS advocates and people with the disease, integrity among doctors and nurses and community workers in the face of frightening unknowns. There has also been bigotry in many forms, political indecision, avoidance of the sharp edge of the realities, and social fragmentation rather than a coming-together. The balance of these elements has led us, repeatedly, one step forward and two steps back, still lacking an effective national AIDS policy that balances fairly the rights of the individual and the protection of the community.

It is not too late to craft that policy, and with it perhaps an important social cohesiveness. From the time we learned that the epidemic was upon us, we had, in truth, our future in our own hands. We need not continue to miss opportunities. We have the power to modify our behavior to protect ourselves and others, to teach our children the realities of the epidemic, to take the public health actions that will benefit the entire community, to see the drug epidemic for what it is: the corrosion of the entire society, and to rouse ourselves to combat it.

For the virus, after all is said and done, is doing the only thing it *can* do—seeking new opportunities to infect individuals, and increasing its own kind.

Though the virus is within the city, we flinch from admitting the deeper reality, all of us: the dragon is within ourselves.

# Bibliography

## Epidemics in History

Camus, Albert, *The Plague* (New York, Random House, 1991). Classic work of fiction/philosophy describing a community's response to the tangible and intangible effects of an epidemic of infectious disease.

Cartwright, Frederick F. in collaboration with Michael D. Biddis, *Disease and History* (New York, Dorset Press, 1972). Analysis of the impact of major historical plagues, beginning in classical times, on political and social trends and events.

Duffy, John, *A History of Public Health in New York City 1625–1966*, Volumes I and II (New York, Russell Sage Foundation, 1968). Traces the history of New York City through the history of its epidemics and emerging public health system.

McNeill, William H., *Plagues and People* (Magnolia, MA, Peter Smith, 1992). Describes the interrelationships of epidemic infectious disease and historical and social processes.

Zinsser, Hans, *Rats, Lice and History* (New York, Bantam Books, 1960). The classic account of the ability of plagues to alter human history.

# Biology of AIDS

*AIDS 1991: A Year in Review* (London: Current Science, 1991). Annual, covering all facets of the epidemic, with especially good material on new knowledge concerning the HIVirus.

Imperato, Pascal James, Ed., *Acquired Immuno-deficiency Syndrome: Current Issues and Scientific Studies* (New York, Plenum Medical Book Company, 1989).

Scientific American Staff, *The Science of AIDS* (New York, W.H. Freeman, 1989). Good general overview of the biological basis of the epidemic.

Volberding, Paul and Mark A. Jacobson, *AIDS Clinical Review 1989* (New York, Marcel Dekker, Inc., 1989).

# AIDS Epidemiology

## International

Miller, Norman and Richard C. Rockwell, Eds., *AIDS in Africa: The Social and Policy Impact,* Volume I in the continuing series, Studies in African Health and Medicine. (Lewiston, The Edwin Mellen Press, 1988).

Pan American Health Organization, *AIDS: Profile of an Epidemic.* Scientific Publication No. 514. (Washington, D.C., 1989).

United Nations and World Health Organization, *Report of the United Nations/World Health Organization Workshop on Modelling the Demographic Impact of the AIDS Epidemic in Pattern II Countries: Progress to Date and Policies for the Future* (New York/Geneva, United Nations/World Health Organization, 1991).

## United States

U.S. Department of Health and Human Services, Public Health Service, *Report of The Surgeon General's Workshop on Children with HIV Infection and Their Families* (DHHS Publication No. HRS-D-MC 87-1, 1987). First overview of the impact of the epidemic on children and families.

Centers for Disease Control, U.S. Department of Health and Human Services, *Reports on AIDS Published in the Morbidity and Mortality Weekly Report,* 1981 through 1992ff (Atlanta). The most critical source for following the pattern of the epidemic. Weekly report on public health issues; this is the standard epidemiologic resource in public health. Most information concerning the spread and understanding of the HIV epidemic appears first in the MMWR.

## New York City

Expert Panel on HIV Seroprevalence Estimates and AIDS Case Projection Methodologies, *Report of the Expert Panel on HIV Seroprevalence Estimates and AIDS Case Projection Methodologies* (New York City Department of Health, 1989). Examination of the methods for estimating the extent of HIV infection and disease in New York City.

New York City Department of Health, *New York City AIDS Case Projections: 1989–1993* (New York, 1989). Standard methodology for estimating future cases of AIDS, using trend lines from previously reported cases.

New York City Department of Health AIDS Surveillance Unit, *AIDS Surveillance Update*, monthly and quarterly, 1983–1992ff (New York). Recurrent monthly series of patterns of AIDS cases in New York.

## AIDS and Society

Abt, Clark C. and Kathleen M. Hardy, Eds., *AIDS and the Courts* (Cambridge, Abt Books Inc., 1990). Discusses legal aspects of the epidemic, including dilemmas of privacy rights and civil liberties.

Andrulis, Dennis P., *Crisis at the Front Line: The Effects of AIDS on Public Hospitals* (New York, Priority Press Publications, 1989). Impact of the epidemic on hospitals: costs, organization, staff.

Bayer, Ronald, *Private Acts, Social Consequences: AIDS and the Politics of Public Health* (New York, The Free Press, 1989). Discussion of social issues raised by the epidemic, with particular stress on dilemmas of protection of society vis-a-vis protection of individual rights, from a bioethical perspective.

Gostin, Larry, *AIDS and the Health Care System* (New Haven, Yale University Press, 1990). Social implications of stresses caused by HIV on the health care system.

Kinsella, James, *Covering the Plague: AIDS and the American Media* (New Brunswick, Rutgers University Press, 1989). Dramatic account of the problems of media coverage of the HIV epidemic.

National Minority AIDS Council, *The Impact of HIV on Communities of Color: A Blueprint for the Nineties* (Washington, D.C., 1992). Advocacy document for focus on HIV and minorities.

Nussbaum, Bruce, *Good Intentions: How Big Business and the Medical Establishment Are Corrupting the Fight Against AIDS* (New York, The Atlantic Monthly Press, 1990). Sensationalist accusé alleging corporate and scientific mismanagement of the fight against HIV.

Presidential Commission on the Human Immunodeficiency Virus Epidemic, *Final Report* (Washington, 1988). First report of the Presidential Commission at close of the Reagan Administration, with series of national recommendations.

Presidential Commission on AIDS, various reports, (Washington, D.C., 1989–1992). Serial report on specific aspects of the epidemic (e.g. AIDS in rural America, AIDS in prisons) by the Bush Administration Presidential Commission.

Price, Monroe Edwin, *Shattered Mirrors: Our Search for Identity and Community in the AIDS Era* (Cambridge, Harvard University Press, 1989). Philosophic discourse on the social "meaning" of the HIV epidemic.

Rogers, David E. and Eli Ginzberg, *Public and Professional Attitudes Toward AIDS Patients: A National Dilemma*, Cornell University Medical College Fifth Conference on Health Policy (Boulder, Westview Press, 1989). Revealing papers concerning the health care impact of professional attitudes toward HIV.

Shilts, Randy, *And the Band Played On: Politics, People, and the AIDS Epidemic* (New York, St. Martin's Press, 1987). The AIDS classic: a journalistic account of the early evolution of the epidemic, with special emphasis on San Francisco.

Sontag, Susan, *Illness As Metaphor,* and *AIDS and its Metaphors* (New York, Anchor Doubleday, 1990). Examines the psychology of epidemics, and the effect that these psychological constructs have upon how we deal with illness.

Wachter, Robert M., *The Fragile Coalition: Scientists, Activists & AIDS* (New York, St. Martin's Press, 1991). Chronicle of the difficult balance necessary to produce the San Francisco International Conference on AIDS, and the tension between science and activism.

## Combating the Epidemic

Arno, Peter S., and K.L. Feiden, *Against the Odds: The Story of AIDS, Drug Development, Politics, and Profits* (New York, HarperCollins, 1992). Narrates the stormy interactions among AIDS advocates, government agencies, and the pharmaceutical industry in the search for treatment.

Institute of Medicine, *Confronting AIDS: Directions for Public Health, Health Care and Research* (Washington, D.C., National Academy Press, 1986). First scientific compilation of a response to the epidemic.

Interagency Task Force on AIDS, *Report to the Mayor* (New York, 1987). Early planning effort by New York City government.

Mayor's Task Force on AIDS, *Assuring Care for New York City's AIDS Population* (New York, 1989). Public-private collaborative effort dealing largely with problem of assuring adequate hospital beds for HIV patients.

Mayor's Task Force on AIDS, *Assuring Care for New York City's AIDS Population. A Fact Book on New York City Hospitals Serving AIDS Patients.* Prepared as an Appendix to the Report of the Mayor's Task Force on AIDS (New York, 1989).

National Research Council, *Evaluating AIDS Prevention Programs*, Susan L. Coyle, Robert F. Boruch, and Charles F. Turner, Eds. (Washington, D.C., National Academy Press, 1989).

National Research Council, *AIDS: Sexual Behavior and Intravenous Drug Use* (Washington, D.C., National Academy Press, 1989).

New York City Department of Health, *HIV Counseling and Testing Policy, March 1987* (New York, 1987). Distributed to all physicians in New York City, describes guidelines for risk assessment, counseling, and testing of patients.

New York City Department of Health, *Guidelines for Physicians on HIV Counseling and Testing and Related Documents* (New York, 1989). Update of the above document, proposes a more proactive and vigorous approach.

New York City Department of Health, *New York City AIDS Task Force Report* (New York, 1989). Five-year strategic plan for resources and services necessary to combat the epidemic in New York City. Produced by a private-public joint task force.

New York City Department of Health, *The Pilot Needle Exchange Study in New York City: A Bridge to Treatment: A Report on the First Ten Months of Operation* (New York, 1989). Reports the operational details and results of the nation's first publicly supported and run needle exchange program.

Norwood, Chris, *Advice for Life: A National Women's Health Network Guide* (New York, Pantheon Books, 1987). First popular account of AIDS prevention from the perspective of women and their risks.

Public Health Service, Department of Health and Human Services, *AIDS: Recommendations and Guidelines: November 1982–November 1986* (Atlanta). Wide-ranging series of guidelines for health professionals and public health departments dealing with the epidemic.

Schinazi, Raymond F. and Andre J. Nahmias, Eds., *AIDS in Children, Adolescents & Heterosexual Adults: An Interdisciplinary Approach to Prevention* (New York, Elsevier, 1988). Papers from the proceedings of a conference that was one of the first devoted to the topic.

Siegel, Larry, Ed., *AIDS and Substance Abuse* (New York, The Haworth Press, 1988). Early analysis, in a series of collected papers, of the public health implications of the connections between AIDS and drugs.

# AIDS Journals

The following are some of the key journals and conference proceedings on AIDS available in medical libraries. Together they form a source for keeping current with scientific developments in the epidemic.

*AIDS*
*AIDS and Public Policy Journal*
*AIDS Care*
*AIDS Literature and News Review*
*AIDS Patient Care*
*ATIN* (AIDS Targeted Information)
International Conferences on AIDS, Programme Abstracts, Published annually, 1985–1992ff.
*Journal of Acquired Immune Deficiency Syndrome*

# Index